How to Deal with Stress and Tension

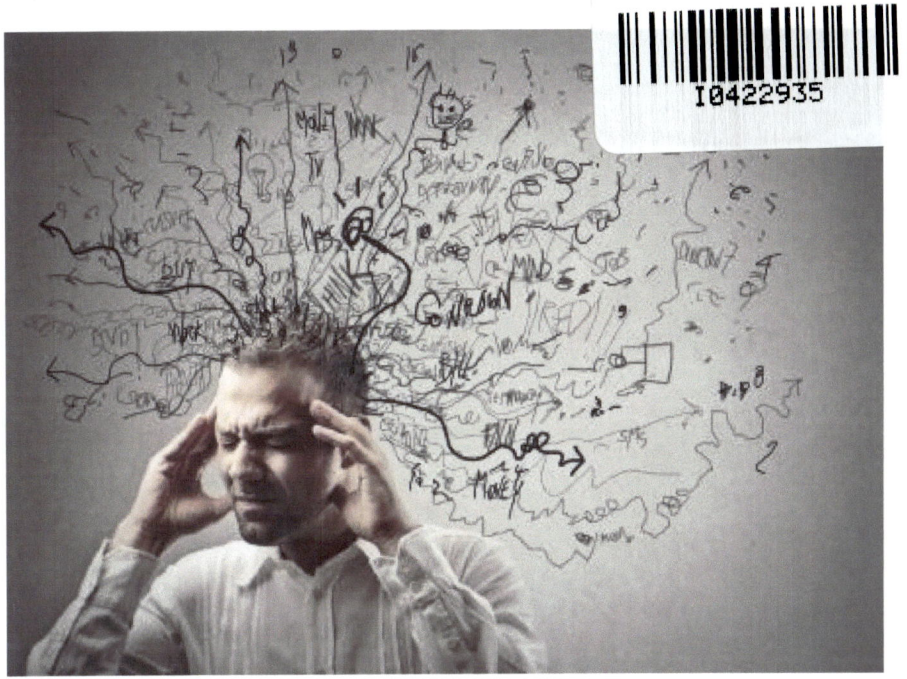

by **Dueep J Singh**

Health Learning Series
Mendon Cottage Books

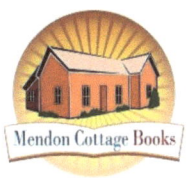

JD-Biz Publishing

Download Free Books!

http://MendonCottageBooks.com

Disclaimer

The information is this book is provided for informational purposes only. It is not intended to be used and medical advice or a substitute for proper medical treatment by a qualified health care provider. The information is believed to be accurate as presented based on research by the author.

The contents have not been evaluated by the U.S. Food and Drug Administration or any other Government or Health Organization and the contents in this book are not to be used to treat cure or prevent disease.

The author or publisher is not responsible for the use or safety of any diet, procedure or treatment mentioned in this book. The author or publisher is not responsible for errors or omissions that may exist.

Warning

The Book is for informational purposes only and before taking on any diet, treatment or medical procedure it is recommended to consult with your primary care provider.

Our books are available at

1. Amazon.com

2. Barnes and Noble

3. Itunes

4. Kobo

5. Smashwords

6. Google Play Books

Table of Contents

Introduction – Why and How Does Stress Affect You? 4

Worrying *About* Stress? Reasons for Stress and Tension 8

Stress Management 13

Work Induced Stress 19

Students and Stress- Study Management 26

Stress and Insomnia 31

Why you should Not Resort to Pills and drugs While Dealing with Stress .36

Yoga – The Best Stress Buster and Meditation 41

Problem-Solving and How That Helps You Cope with Stress 46

What are the things I cannot help?..49

What are the things that I can solve? 49

Conclusion 53

Author Bio..55

Publisher...66

Introduction – Why and How Does Stress Affect You?

Do you suffer from stress and tension? The reason you are reading this e-book shows that you believe that you may be suffering from stress, you want to know all about how you can get rid of stress, or better still, you want to know how you can prevent stress from influencing your life and lifestyle.

Well, this book is going to give you plenty of tips and techniques on how you can cope with stress, reasons for why you suffer from stress, how to prevent stress as a student, or in the office, stress management, and other factors related to stress and tension.

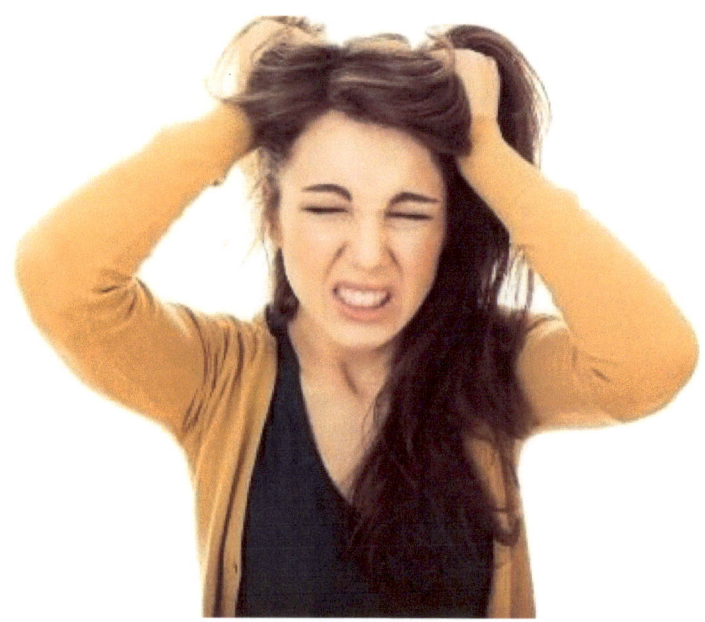

Remember that a little bit of stress and anxiety is part and parcel of everybody's daily life. We can just call it thinking about day to day worries and trivial problems. On the other hand, when these problems are blown up to such an extent, that we think that we cannot solve them, we cannot bear them, and we just do not know what to do about them, we have reached the stress and tension stage. That is when the mind has begun to worry whether it can take on the burden and responsibility of solving a supposedly insurmountable problem. And then the mind says, "no, sorry, just cannot do it." But it has to be done. And so you get stressed.

Now let us come to why your mind immediately said, "*No, sorry, just cannot do it.* You just have to cope some other way. Put it on the back burner for now." This is one of the natural defensive tactics built in a thinking brain. It is always going to take the easy way out, in order not to burden itself with something which it knows through experience, is going to cause it problems, hassles and future tension. And so the mind tries to pretend that this problem does not exist.

It wants you to believe that if you ignore the problem, it will go away. But the problem is still there, lurking in some form, and you will have to face it someday. So if you have a really strong willpower and mind, you face the problem. Once you face it, you find that it definitely was not a mountain, which your mind had made. It was just a itty bitty molehill.

Now let me give you an example. I got my driving license, when I was 18 and learned how to drive a really heavy car – a 270 HP Ambassador. It was a really powerful machine and subconsciously my mind "decided" that I could not control it, and I was not a good enough driver to control that lean, mean, sleek machine. So I started getting stressed whenever I had to drive it or anything else. That was because my mind was influencing me and making me believe that I was not capable of managing a car.

This sort of subtle influence reached such stress making stages that I stopped driving completely. And also, I did not notice but I had started feeling afraid of driving *any vehicle*, because that subconscious command of all vehicles are dangerous, so better not drive them, had permeated through my mind. So in order to prevent stress and tension, I never drove anything on the roads for the next two decades, relying on public transport to get me to and from my destinations.

And then came a time when I had to buy a vehicle, which I did with fear and trembling. It was just a Honda scooter. Now this was a simple two wheeler. But my mind had made it into a dangerous thing, and I, who considered myself a strong firm adult was afraid of driving it! So I got stressed whenever I was on the road, because my mind kept telling me, "it is dangerous, it is dangerous" and subconsciously I had begun to believe that I would meet with an accident, because I could not drive properly and control it. In reality, I am a very good and safe driver. But see how stress had made me question my own judgment and capacities. This is how one's mind influences you.

And then something else happened, which is the perfect classic example of a psychological state of how you can deal with stress and how once your mind accepts a fact, stress and tension is removed in a moment.

A couple of weeks after I had bought that Scooter, I had to drive somebody to the hospital in a car. I had not driven for 25 years. But I did not allow that particular stress inducing item to impinge on my conscious mind because I was stressed out for another major top priority reason – get the patient to the nearest hospital ASAP. And I drove the heavy, unwieldy car with the patient to the hospital, – only to find out that he was just suffering from indigestion and not a possible heart attack – and that relief in itself was epiphany enough; Sudden and striking moment of mental revelation.

It was only when I sat back on my chair totally unstressed and free of tension that I began to notice that hey, what was the big deal? I had faced my fear of driving cars. They were just pieces of machinery which I could control. So what was so frightening about a little itty bitty scooter? If it was going to make me stressed out and tense, I would be rather stupid, would not I? And why had I prevented myself for two decades from enjoying my life thoroughly, just I and my Ambassador going around the compass? I had created a needless aura of stress, fear and tension in myself and wasted so much precious time, instead of facing this fear straight in the eye.

Needless to say, now I drive all over the place, mountains and plains, with absolutely no stress, tension, or worry about my not being able to control my vehicle ever.

So now that you know how stress affects you, here are many tips and techniques, starting with facing the reason plainly and getting your mind to accept that. Your mind will go in for line of least resistance, and your body is going to follow suit. So once we learn how to tackle stress, we will also learn how to cope with it.

Apart from mental fatigue, a state of chronic stress is also going to have a physical impact on your state of good health and well-being. You may neglect eating food thus directly affecting your health. People suffering from stress also suffer from high blood pressure, ulcers, and tension induced diseases. Now, this happens to be a vicious circle. You are stressed because you are ill. You are ill, and that causes you stress. This is a no-win situation both ways.

Worrying *About* Stress? Reasons for Stress and Tension

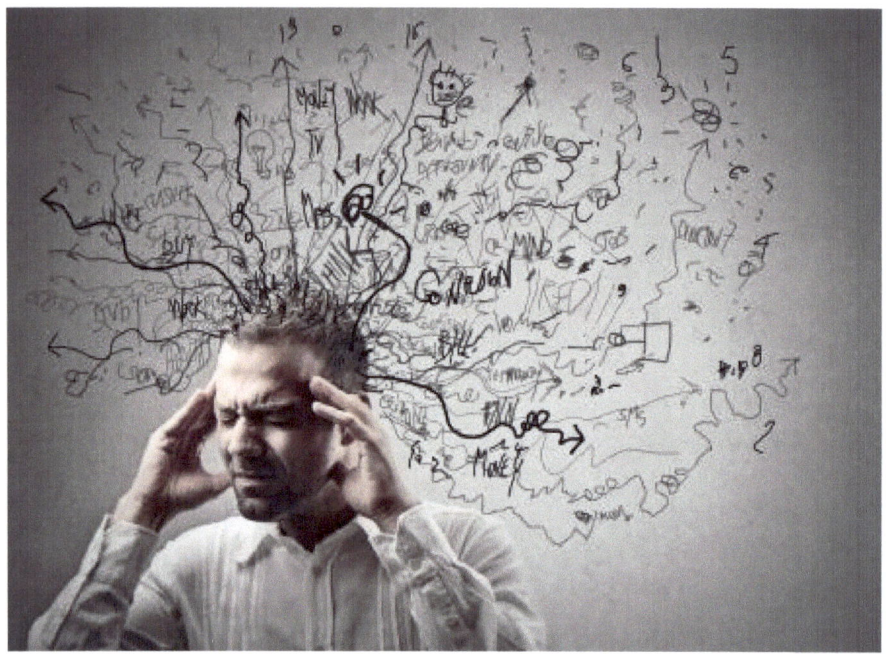

Have you reached a stage in your life when you think that whatever you are doing is not worth doing and how best you need to get out of it, and you cannot get out of it, and what are you going to do now? And all this thought is causing you a major headache? And then some well-wisher comes around to tell you that you look stressed. The moment you hear the word "stress" you immediately start worrying about whether you are stressed or not! There are many reasons why you may be suffering from stress and tension. Chronic stress occurs only when you find yourself worrying about some point which you think you cannot solve. It starts the moment you wake up.

You immediately begin to think about how to solve that particular problem. You spend your time thinking about how to solve that particular problem. You get stressed out. Notice that you are not making any efforts into taking concrete steps to solve that particular problem. *You are just thinking about how to solve it.* And then you get stressed, because you not know how to solve it. And then you find yourself undergoing these symptoms –

- Intense fatigue.
- Loss of concentration
- Irritated and grumpy behavior.
- No interest in your surroundings.
- Loss of appetite
- Feeling that you have to do something. But you do not know where to start.
- Feeling that all the problems you have to face are beyond your capacity to solve or tackle.
- Wanting support from somebody who is going to solve all your problems.
- Getting into self-pitying mode by associating and linking your problems with someone else's behavior or shortcomings.
- Blaming someone else for all your problems and feeling depressed.
- Feeling that nothing is worth it.

  Now, this last one is one symptom of stress and tension, which needs immediate attention. All the rest are part and parcel of stress and tension, but the moment you fear that things are beyond you and that you may take drastic steps to solve them – yes, stressed people commit suicide very often over matters which they think beyond their control. – And that is why it is necessary to understand the factors which contribute to your high stress levels.

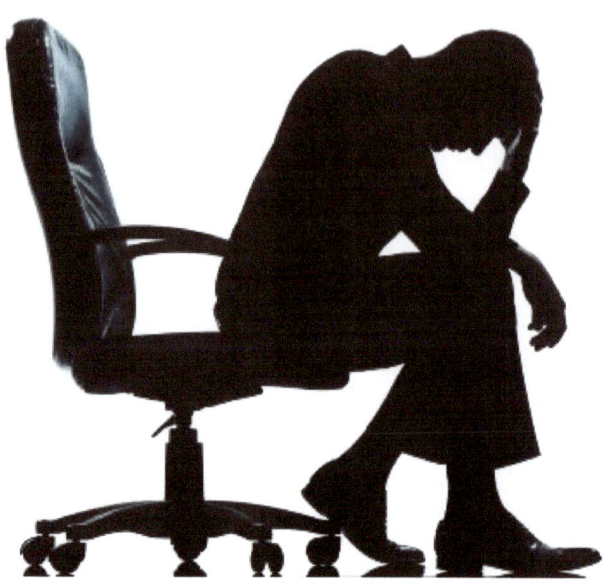

How do I cope with everything piled on me all at once?

Did you know that the majority of people out there suffer from some form or other of stress? That can be seen when they feel depressed and miserable. If you find somebody around you who is pessimistic, tells you that he cannot do something, he thinks some problem beyond his problem-solving capacities and capabilities, well, he is well on his way to being a stressed person. If you are not one, but recognize these symptoms in somebody you know, understand that he may be stressed. Chronic stress and tension can lead to an even worse condition – chronic depression. So if you do not recognize the symptoms of stress, you may find yourself a victim of depression later. You can manage to pull out of stress and tension with a little bit of effort, enthusiasm, dedication, willpower and support. People who are depressed normally do not manage to get back into their normal state of good health, optimism, cheer, confidence, positivity, and assurance.

So you find yourself worrying just because somebody inquired whether you are stressed and you decided to spend some time wondering whether you really were stressed and is it showing in your general behavior and on your face, snap out of it right now. You really cannot afford to start worrying about whether you are really stressed and whether it is one of the major factors which are causing you stress and tension!

There are so many other reasons out there which may be contributing factors for tension, worry and stress. Many of them include financial, emotional, personal and professional factors.

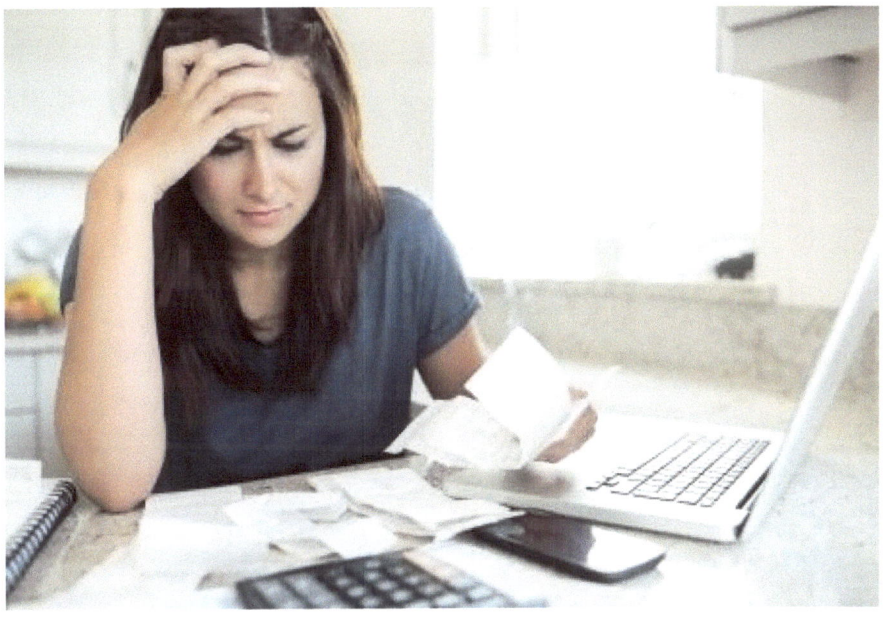

Stressing yourself out on things which may never happen is one of the reasons why so many people get stressed, thanks to their overactive imagination.

Fear is a contributing factor for stress. You may be stressed because you are worried about job security, and whether you have enough of finances in case you are given the pink slip. Well, here you are, worrying yourself needlessly about something which has not happened and which will never happen. You have contributed a lot to unnecessary baggage on your brain. Now this is not a very healthy activity for your mind, brain, soul and spirit. So when your brain goes into overload mode, it is going to stress out and say "enough is enough. I really, really cannot take on all these problems, which I have to solve." And that is when you find yourself in dire stressed straits.

So unless the reason is valid, justified, and present right at the moment and not a figment of your imagination, try hard to persuade your brain not to get stressed. That is going to be much better for you in the long run.

Stress Management

Do you find yourself irritated at tiny things? Do you find yourself extremely tired mentally and physically? Do you find yourself incapable of doing even the most easy of tasks at home or in the office? Do you find yourself frazzled at the end of the day? Is it quite impossible for you to relax even after the day's work is done because you are worrying about tomorrow? Do you find yourself unable to concentrate and feel that your brain has turned into mush and cotton wool?

These are just some common symptoms of stress. So if you find yourself getting overly anxious, mentally, it is going to have a detrimental effect upon your physical being. You can consider yourself to be in the stressed-out category. A little bit of stress and strain is normal, but being stressed-out is definitely not desirable or advisable.

Here are some very easy to implement stress management tips, which you can use to reduce stress in the office. First of all recognize that you are feeling stressed. You find yourself gritting your teeth, you feel a dull pounding in your temples, your shoulder muscles and neck muscles have started to pain you, and you feel like exploding in a bad temper. The moment you recognize these stress symptoms, say loudly to yourself, "I am stressed. I need to relax. Nothing is so important as cannot be done in a few minutes after I am relaxed." Take deep breaths , and look out of the window to some pleasant green vista. Do not have time to look out of the window, you say? Make some time! Or have pleasant scenery placed in a prominent place right in front of your desk.

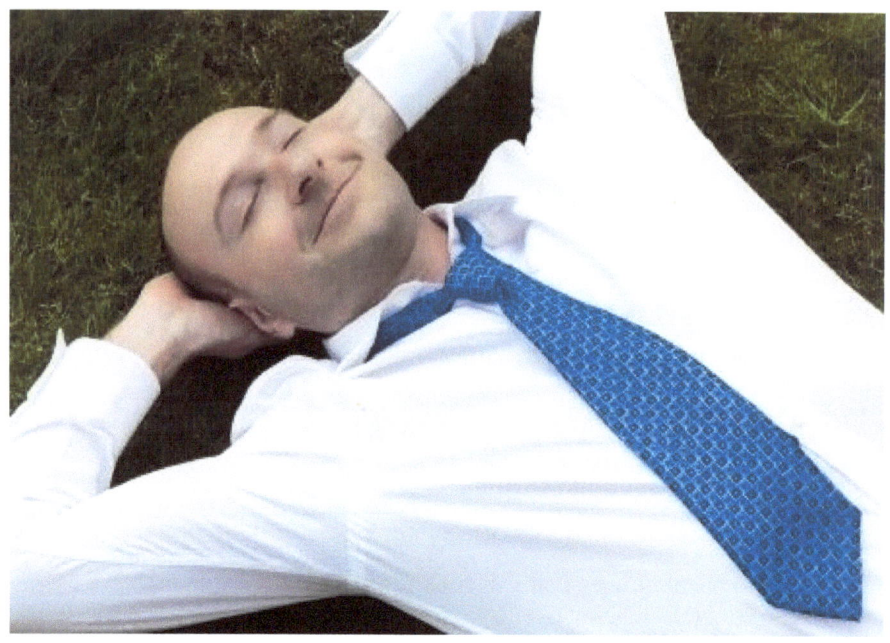

If you are at home, and you find yourself stressed while doing something, just get up and move around the room. Take deep breaths. You may want to go into the kitchen and make a loud noise clanking pots and pans together while washing them. I find getting under a shower and just making a throaty grrrrrrrrrrrrrrrrrrrrrrr noise works wonders! Emulate a bee trapped in an envelope. Consider yourself of being in such a situation. Make a noise to reduce the tension knotting your neck and shoulder muscles. And then come out of the bath refreshed in order to tackle your stress causing problems again.

And then follow the given steps –

Prioritize your tasks. Everything cannot be done like right now. So, write down the tasks, which take top priority on your "have to be done" scale. You are going to be surprised to see that this stress management tip of making a list of all your priorities calms you down, because you are doing something positive and constructive. So, now that you have written down the priority list, start completing the tasks from the top of the list. Number one is what needs to be done first and so on and so forth.

Delegate some authority to somebody else. Do not take on too much responsibility on yourself, especially by saying yes to everybody who asks you to do them a favor, please. You may be gaining brownie points in the office hierarchy but you have absolutely no time to yourself or to relax.

You are going to find yourself stressed out, while other people take it cool.

Remember to spend at least 10 to 15 minutes of your day in fresh air, without access to your cell phone or to your computer. When I suggested this way of relaxing to a stressed-out person, he said rather proudly, "Who has time to relax, I am so busy that I need to be in touch with everybody who wants to get in touch with me to solve some problems popping up in the office."

I did not tell this person that he was trying to prove to himself that he was so important and indispensable that nobody could do without him. He would stress himself out trying to believe this fact and not relaxing. On the other hand, if he was really so indispensable, holding the reins of his office in his own two hands without delegating any authority to anybody else, it was a given that when he went down due to a stress induced heart attack or stroke, his office would be in chaos, because there was nobody with authority, initiative, and the common sense needed to make a final decision for the good of the business or for their own good.

Well, he was digging his own pitfall. Such people love the idea that they are stressed because they are so important. It gives them a high! Well, I hope you are not one of them!

Concentrate on just one task at a time; Multi-taskers find themselves subject to stress, more than the plodders, concentrating on one task at a time. You might want to make a list of some things which can be done later.

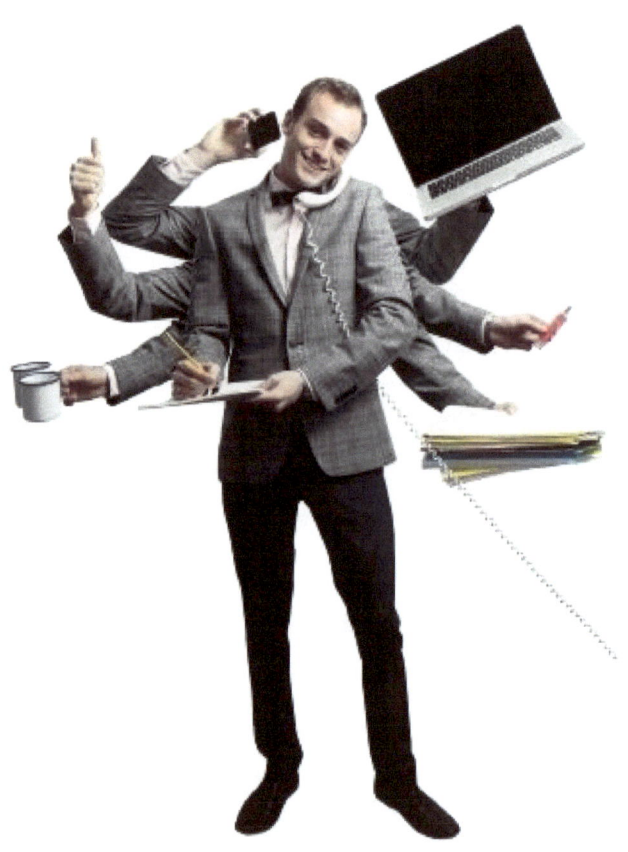

Are you a multi-tasker? There are some people who thrive on multitasking. They just enjoy doing 13 things at one time. They say they find it, mentally and physically challenging and stimulating. They are also going to be the ones who are going to burn out physically and mentally within a couple of years, because as their body slows down due to age, their mind is going to say "of course you can do that, you could do that 10 years ago." And then the mind is going to get stressed, because these overachievers think that there is something wrong with them, because they could not keep up to their levels of high achievement. That is why you need to understand that ambition is one of the reasons why so many people are stressed out. Also, they compete with the Joneses, subconsciously, 24 x 7. These people will never learn the first rule of no stress – you owe it to yourself to take care of you. Nobody is going to do it for you

So if you are proud to be a multi-tasker, now, teach yourself to take it slow. Nobody is going to give you a prize if you exhaust yourself acting a busy bee. If you want to show off your multitasking skills and impress the people around you, well, that is your prerogative. They may praise you initially. But on the other hand, they may begin to think that it is possible that you are showing them up, especially when you prove to them that they cannot do everything which you do.

Believe me, anybody who has done a job successfully cannot resist crowing about it. You have done that, I have done that. If it was worth doing, and garnered praise, it was a job well done. On the other hand, if we kept on harping on how well we could do that job, we would be ourselves creating an atmosphere of stress and tension around ourselves. Our neighbors, friends, colleagues, family members, employees, and employers would begin to think us tiresome bores. They would get stressed out, because they were not as efficient as you. You would get stressed out because they would show this reaction in their body language and in their interaction with you. So unless you are completely hippopotamus skinned and could not care less about the people around you and their reactions, try not to induce a stress filled atmosphere in your vicinity. This is a matter of common human psychology.

Work Induced Stress

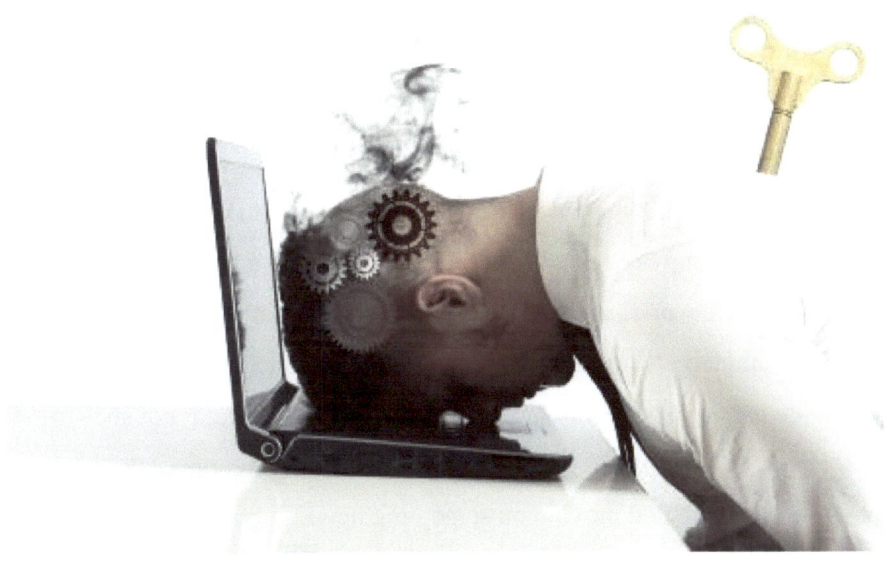

My job wound me up and now my springs are broken and my cogwheels rusted...

If the idea of waking up and going to work every morning instinctively makes you cringe, one major stress factor and source is in your office itself. It might be a colleague, it might be a superior who is causing you to feel that you cannot face just another day in paradise in the company of that horrible XYZ.

Somebody once asked me how I managed to juggle so many career options throughout my life, enjoying each one of them, and not getting stressed? I should have been completely burned out by now, which unfortunately is the case of *all* of my friends, colleagues and acquaintances who started out their careers when I did. They are very successful, many of them in top level envy making positions, very well-known and prosperous. And all of them suffer from plenty of health problems induced by stress brought on by family and professional problems. How come I had managed to survive all that to my 40s without an ensuing burnout?

I told them that, first of all, I enjoyed what I did. I never went in for another career change, without an interest in it. Also, I liked working, burnishing my skills, gaining knowledge and experience and earning a honest day's pay for an honest day's work but I was not an obsessive workaholic. I had not set out goals and targets for myself which I had to complete within the next five years slaving at just one job. And that is the reason why I did not stick to one career, but had plenty of fun searching for other career options, getting proficient in them and moving on something new.

Also, I did just that amount of work throughout the day, which was within my capacity and capabilities. I knew exactly how much to push myself without getting physically, mentally and spiritually exhausted. And the day I began to feel stressed in a monotonous job and started bringing my worries back home with me, I began to look for another change.

I am lucky here I got a chance to forge my own path through life marching to my own drummer. But that unfortunately is not the option for a majority of us, because we have responsibilities and commitments and just cannot up and leave. How many of us face an unpleasant atmosphere in the home, office, school or anywhere else because we are stuck there. We cannot get out. Even though our jobs are stress filled and also they are causing us incipient ulcers at the old age of 30, we need the job to pay our bills and to pay off mortgages, loans, and other burdens we took unto ourselves voluntarily or out of sheer necessity. So we need to know everything about stress management in such cases.

The easiest stress management tip is to identify the cause of stress and make alternative arrangements to get rid of that particular problem in an effective manner.

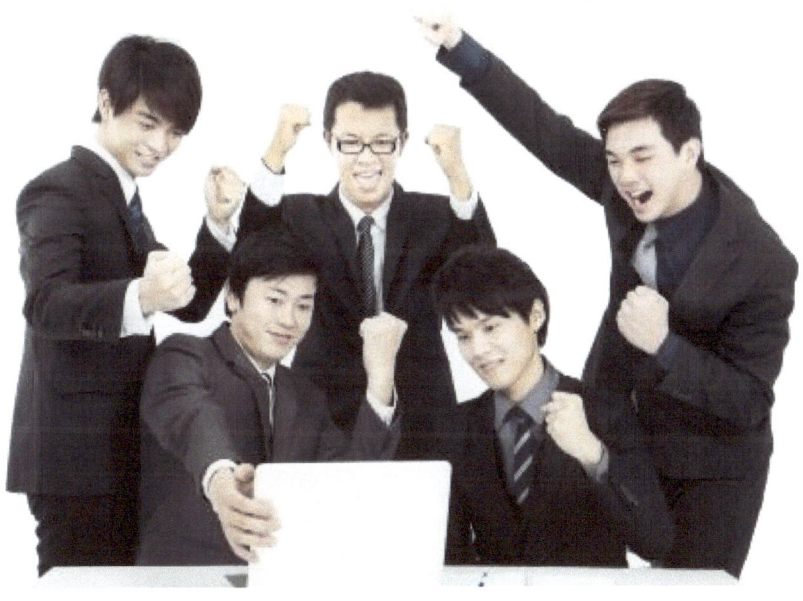

A harmonious and pleasant atmosphere in the office is conducive to less stress...

So, what can be considered the common sources of stress at work? Many people suffering from stress, which is due to causes in the office definitely do not talk it out, because they are too shy to do so, they think they will be ridiculed. Or they are too worried about losing their jobs. That in itself is one major source of stress, job security, scary enough to give you sleepless nights.

If it is a colleague, the easiest stress management tip to meet with this problem is a direct face-to-face confrontation putting all the cards on the table, with an umpire to monitor the proceedings. You might want to talk things over with the colleague, asking him what his problem is. Once people get to know that you are facing a problem with some particular issue in the office, it is going to make your workplace environment much more congenial and easy to live in.

You are stressed out, because you have taken up many commitments, which you need to fulfill before a deadline? Learn to say no. This is going to reduce the work pressure on you. That is the best stress management tip. It is also going to help you a lot in your personal life too!

One fine evening I was winding up my work for the day, when I noticed a colleague G. who I had invited for an after work snack in our favorite snack bar say, "no, you go, I have to do some work." I found that G. had taken on someone else's work, because that particular colleague K. had this persuasive way of cajoling someone to take on some of her duties. And this particular colleague of mine was too gentle a person and could not say no when somebody said, "You are my friend, please could you do this for me I would be so grateful to you" in a melting tone. I soon found out that this particular shirker managed to get most of her work done by other people, but she took all the credit and the kudos. So this once I was going to make sure that my susceptible to cajolement friend was not going to be a workhorse.

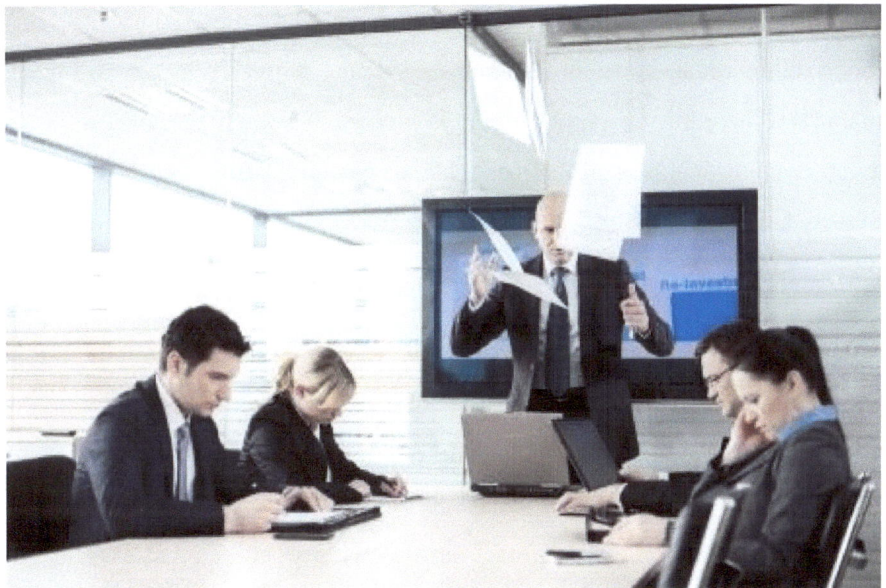

"Do you know how to do the work which K. has asked you to complete?"

My friend did not know how to do that. But she said that K. had said that it would be a really good learning experience for G! Now here was a relative newcomer in our office being imposed upon by a chronic shirker. I knew what was going to happen next. K would praise her to the earth. She really, really did a good job. And poor G would soon find herself doing her work as well as K's work and getting to be really stressed in the bargain.

So I decided to give both of them a helping hand.

I told G that she just had to type in the data which I would dictate to her. She did so. And she fed in the previous year's data, including financial details and statistics given to her by me. K, breezing in early the next morning, said four or five thank you's to G, and went off to give her report with obsolete outdated data. And then, as expected, she came back red-faced – after a right royal expected ticking off – and shouting at G for messing up her report. G put on an innocent face and said, "Your report? Why would I want to make *your* report for you? Is not that your job?" With the whole office and the senior members of the management listening avidly to this washing of dirty laundry in public. The result was that K was asked politely to look for another job after the senior management found out how she got her work done by other people at least 65% of the time.

Moral of the story is – you may hoodwink many people, most of the time, but you have to get ready for being exposed publicly, especially when you find yourself confronted with insouciant troubleshooters like I always ready to make mischief in order to protect our friends from potential stress and tension!

Now this is a piece of office politics, which many people may face when they work in an office. And this is why you may find yourself stressed out.

But, you say, "Forget about other people's work, I cannot manage to finish my own work within the given time limit. And that is stressing me!"

Well, I sympathize with you here, because I have been there seen that. In fact, there were times when I had a deadline and found myself dreaming up the stages of work, which I had done previously, which I had missed, and which needed to be done. Talk about nightmares! This happens when your brain is so busy worrying, that it cannot let go and relax. This is the first stage of incipient stress.

People who are stressed out because they do not seem to have enough time to complete all their work need to understand one formula -- effective stress management is done through effective time management. If you are stressed just because you cannot reach the office in time, why did you not/can you not get out of the house half an hour early? Effective time management is going to help you have time to do your work effectively, instead of piling on the stress, while multitasking.

Students and Stress- Study Management

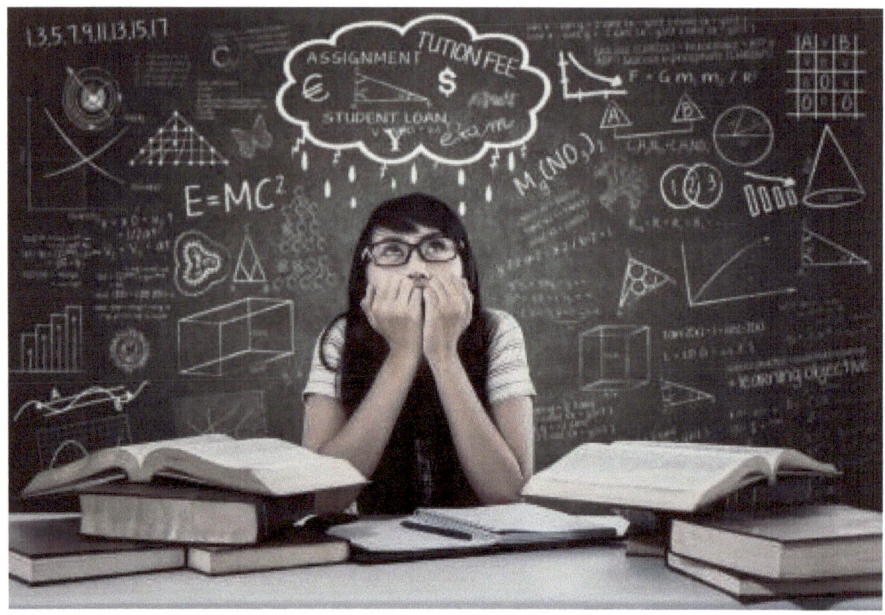

Did you know that a large percentage of people suffering from stress are students? That is because as I said before, they have taken on a responsibility to achieve some particular goal within a given period of time. And that is why they spend a lot of their time burning the midnight oil. They have not learned the subtle art of study management when related to stress management.

When do most students suffer from stress? Some of them start suffering from stress right at the beginning of their academic year. These are students who are result driven. Others face temporary bouts of stress periodically especially around exam time. That is because they have not learned the first rules of study management when related to stress management.

So how do you keep study management and stress management in its proper perspective?

Stress in small doses definitely does not hurt you, because it keeps you on your toes, but if you find yourself being overwhelmed with stress, because of study responsibility, an examination coming on, papers to be given before the end of the week, or any other reason, you need to sit back and put things in their proper perspective.

Now, anybody who is under the impression that he does not have time to relax is just asking for those tense muscles and clenched teeth at the end of the day. Positive thinking is definitely one goal, which you must try to achieve, and the moment you find yourself slipping back into the morass of "I really cannot," you need to pull yourself up and give yourself a firm talking to. In fact, this is the time, when you would need a little bit of humor, especially if you call yourself a limp, spineless, Jell-O packed primitive ectoplasm, who needs to become a positive thinking human right away. These descriptions would be quite enough to make you smile, and once you relax, you are going to find that things are looking better.

I remember a time when I was studying for my Degree. I was not really serious about getting top grade marks, because I did not intend to become a lecturer or an academician at that stage. I knew all I had to do was sit with my books in a concentrated eight-hour sitting for two days and assimilate the whole course taught during the year.

I was fortunate that way to have such powers of concentration and assimilation, and that is why I never felt stressed while collecting my myriad graduate and postgraduate degrees. Because study for me was fun and interesting, instead of being a burden and a duty. But for most of the stressed-out students out there, study is something which has to be done and it takes on the onerous shape of a painful burden. And that is why they find themselves being stressed. My classmates and roommates on the other hand, went into jitters at the mere thought of exams looming in front of them. And they studied nights and day in day out without taking time out to eat or drink, or to have a breath of fresh air. So by the time they were ready to give their exams, they were totally mentally and physically exhausted. They were just running on caffeine and adrenaline. And the moment they had finished writing their papers, all that knowledge was wiped clean out of their overburdened brains.

So can you understand the reason why they were stressed-out and why I did not face such a problem? I never thought studied to be a reason for stress. I took interest in the subjects which I was studying. I read a paragraph, and then closed my eyes, and made my brain understand the knowledge which was being imparted to me. Now that knowledge was solid. My friends on the other hand, were just studying by rote without their brains really taking in the knowledge. So one word or thought process missed somewhere, and the brain would seize up – "what happens then, I cannot remember." No wonder they were stressed-out.

Stress when taken to extremes, especially when you find yourself losing touch with reality, friends, and things you would enjoy, in a normal state of mind, it is time to get things in proper perspective and priority mode.

1. Are you sleeping badly?
2. Did you miss out on any meals?
3. Did you miss going out in the fresh air for the past couple of days?

4. Have you been sitting in front of the console for the past 3 hours without a break?
5. Do you snap at the people around you?
6. Are you feeling depressed, and distressed?

If the answer to any or all of these is yes, it is time to snap out of it and fast. These are the incipient symptoms of prolonged and possibly chronic stress. These symptoms are going to interfere with your health, your studies, and the overall quality of your life. So, now that you are a responsible student, you need to see how you can manage stress, especially when it is study induced, and in such a manner that you do not find yourself jumping from one state of crisis to another.

People who do not like to exercise that definitely going to have an excuse that they are studying. But the moment you get those endorphins and blood corpuscles moving, the more energetic you are going to feel. So remember to try out some short energetic bursts of activity, even if it is standing up and touching your toes, after a given period of study. You will also find yourself sleeping better at the end of the day.

Do not miss out on any meals, because starving your body of the necessary grains, cereals, proteins, fruit, vegetables and nuts is not a good idea. And it is definitely not going to help you lose weight, either. Also try to avoid caffeine, chocolate, sugary food, alcohol, drugs (unless prescribed by a doctor), and junk food. Do not eat and study simultaneously. Eating is relaxation time. Take some time out to communicate with the rest of your friends, because that is the best way of relaxing. You might want to start up a study group with your friends, which means rest and relaxation as well as studying.

Make a daily planner, which is going to help you get through your priorities. And then concentrate on completing those priorities first. You might want to spread the major time-consuming activities into small chunks of half an hour a day over a number of days. Take help from your advisers, lecturers, friends, tutors, and everybody who can help you out. And definitely do not tire yourself out. Unwind with music, a shower, and reading some light fiction. Remember to keep your proper perspective -- a good grade does not automatically mean automatic happiness and future career success. Be a good enough student, and that is going to be good enough for everybody around you. Be realistic in your expectations.

Stress and Insomnia

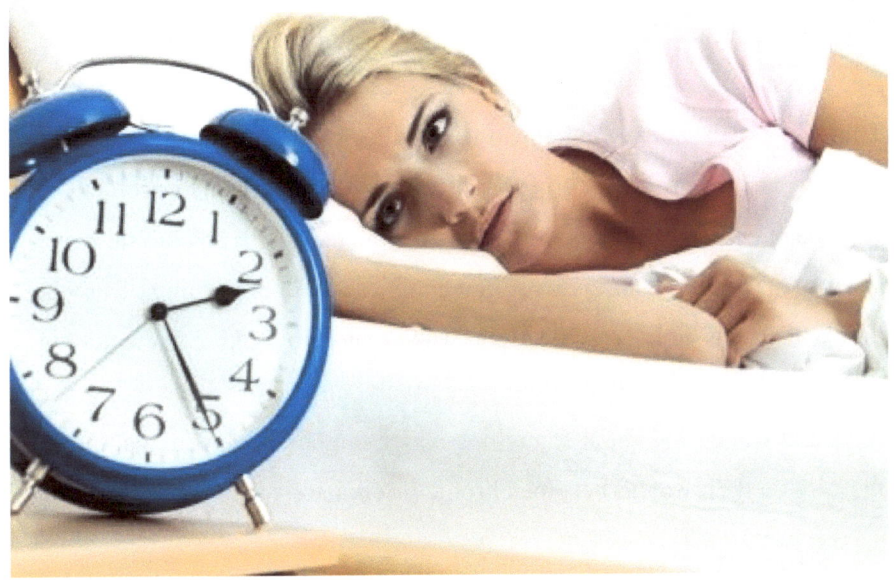

Is that you worried and unable to sleep?

A stressed-out colleague once told me that he was rather worried because he was suffering from insomnia. And he was getting more stressed-out, because he was suffering from insomnia.

Now this is an occupational hazard with stressed-out people. They are stressed because of their problems. They cannot sleep because they are worrying about how to solve their problems. They start suffering from insomnia. And then they get stressed out, because they cannot sleep and rest properly. They feel tired because they cannot sleep well. They then get more stressed because they are not sleeping well. Well this is a continuous vicious cycle, and if you find yourself suffering from stress-induced insomnia here are some tips and techniques which can help you relax and get rid of one of the factors causing you insomnia.

Many of us suffer from what is called white nights when you cannot go to sleep even when you happen to be relaxed as snug as a bug in your rug. This might be because you happen to be suffering from tension, anxiety about work, health, job security, family, business, or any other problem which can cause you an anxiety. Some people happen to be chronic worry warts, who positively enjoy worrying about each and everything. But when they extend this activity to the night, when they start looking at the ceiling and keeping awake at night, thinking actively, instead of letting their mind relax and wondering about something which might not happen, that means they are on their way to become chronic insomniacs.

The symptoms of severe insomnia happen to be a complete inability to go to sleep at your regular sleeping time. Even if you manage to get up to sleep, you find yourself waking up and then spend the next couple of hours thinking of nothing much, counting sheep, thinking about what you need to do tomorrow, thinking about that hard-hitting, to the point retort that you should have said to XYZ to show him/her that you were not a walkover/doormat , and so there. [This last activity normally comes to our mind at 3 o'clock in the morning of a sleepless night, and is about seven hours too late to have made a really lasting and powerful impression. But that is the way the cookie crumbles, no pun intended.]

Not even a glass of hot milk and honey can make you go to sleep again. So if you want to ensure that you do not suffer from insomnia brought about by stress, try these relaxation steps right now.

If you are a worry wart, be like Scarlett O'Hara. Tell yourself that you are going to make all your decisions tomorrow. The moment you start thinking about by worry making problems again, repeat the Scarlett O'Hara aphorism, very firmly yet once again. Your brain will need this firm talking to a couple of times, before it decides that you really do not want to think about your problems which are causing you stress and which are preventing you from going to sleep

To make sure that you do not suffer from insomnia over again, try these easy to implement tips right now.

•   Have a light meal two hours before you go to sleep. Many of us have a very heavy dinner with plenty of alcohol, and cheese and wonder why we cannot find it easy to go to sleep. It is true that rich people during Regency times had 8 course meals, but they also spent the rest of the time dancing during the party following. They also exercised regularly and partied late into the night after their heavy meals. However, they went to bed early in the morning, after plenty of dancing, and woke up in the afternoon. So they had plenty of time for the meal to digest at least partially before they went to sleep. Besides this, they were completely tired out and never forced themselves to stay awake. So they definitely did not suffer from insomnia ever.

Going too soon to bed after eating a heavy dinner is tantamount to inviting indigestion and heartburn. So, if you do not go for à walk after dinner, you won't be able to be tired enough to go to sleep. Do not go energetic disco dancing after a very heavy meal. We do not have the constitutions of boa constrictors, and thus we cannot manage heavy meals, along with heavy exercise at the same time. So restrict yourself to just one languid leisurely meandering through the daisies walk after dinner.

• Don't eat sitting in front of the idiot box. The eating posture is so bad that your stomach is slumped. The idea of eating at a dining table meant sitting up straight in a good chair and eating your food slowly. TV dinners are one of the main causes of insomnia, because they are eaten at a gallop, in a slouched position, and then one goes to bed soon after the movie is finished.

• You may find yourself suffering from insomnia the older you get due to a change in sleep patterns. You might not be able to sleep, in such a restful manner, and find yourself undergoing even more white nights. You will find it easier to wake up earlier in the morning even though you find yourself more sleepy from the evenings itself. So remember down to stress yourself out if you are in your 50s, and find yourself waking up earlier than normal. If your body is rested and relaxed, it knows that it has had enough sleep.

• If you remember to keep yourself mentally and physically busy, it is very easy for you to go to sleep easily. This is what is known as healthy tiredness. However, if you happen to have plenty of free time, and you find yourself drinking more coffee and alcohol as a result of this free time, you are going to suffer from insomnia. These food items are conducive to making sure that you have been a complete white night. That is the reason why coffee is drunk while you are completing a project which needs to be done now, and you are not allowed time to sleep!

• If you happen to be suffering from chronic pain caused by some disease like cancer, arthritis or even pain in the back, you will find it very difficult to go to sleep. The medications given for the alleviation of this pain is enough to make you keep awake also. Also, these are the major reasons for stress, because you know you are suffering from a disease, you cannot help it, and this feeling of helplessness is aggravating your mental and physical stress condition.

If you find yourself stressed and tense and unable to sleep because of depression and anxiety, you need to consult your doctor as soon as possible. He's going to look at your symptoms and then prescribe suitable therapies, so that you can find it easier to sleep. Some of the most popular behavioral therapies are all about changing your sleep patterns by practicing a behavior which is more conducive to a good night's rest. Relaxing, listening to music, unwinding two hours before going to sleep, taking walks, exercises, having a hot bath, having hot milky drinks before you put to sleep are part and parcel of behavioral treatments. Many doctors have decided that such treatments are more effective and better than giving medication for sleep to their patients.

Why you should Not Resort to Pills and drugs While Dealing with Stress

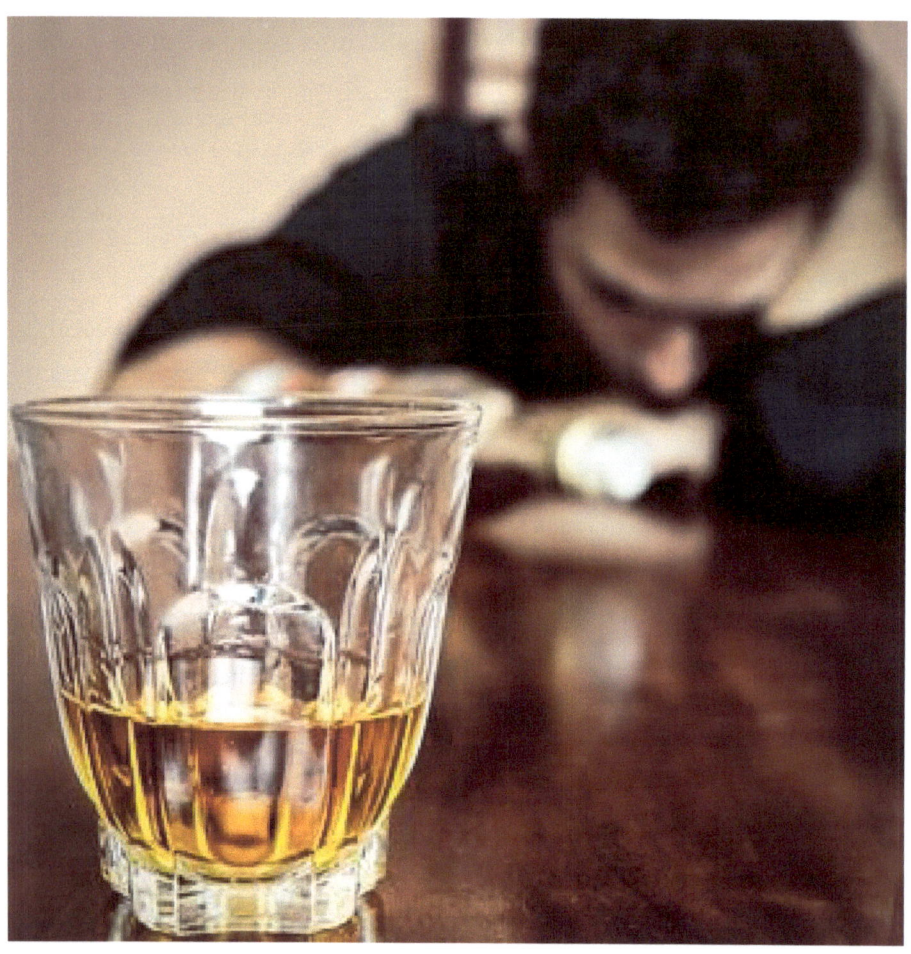

I have found a number of acquaintances suffering from stress popping pills. According to them, this is a good way to deal with stress. I think this taking of drugs is not advisable.

Some doctors may prescribe some drugs, if you are suffering from insomnia in order to make you relax. You can take prescribed sleeping drugs to try to get to sleep, because after all, you need to concentrate on how to get a healthy night's sleep but it is much better to get along without their help. Many of these drugs cause dependency upon them, even though they happen to be in very small doses. Even after you have been cured of insomnia, you want to take those drugs to go to sleep. Some of these prescribed medicines also have side effects like edema and allergy. You might also find yourself sleepwalking after you have taken some of these drugs! That is the reason why doctors do not let you take these drugs for more than a couple of days. Your job is to make sure you go to sleep without the help of any of these drugs so that future drug dependency should not ever be an issue in question here.

Why do I not advise pills as a stress buster and a means of relieving stress? Remember that most of the people that we get out there are to cure our bodies of sickness. A doctor prescribing a patient to take a course of medicine is intended on curing his problem. He knows that taking such medicine may have a long-term side effect , especially if it has been taken over a long period of time. That is because the body has changed its biological, bio-physiological and natural system in order to incorporate with the healing properties of the drug, which after all is a foreign body. Nevertheless, his first duty is to make sure that the body is cured of the infection. That is going to happen with the help of the prescribed drug. After that, he is going to give you more drugs to counteract the side effects caused by the prolonged taking of the previous drug. And that drug is going to have even more side effects.

Do you know that is the reason why so many people are addicted to drugs which were prescribed to them to reduce pain or some other symptoms of diseases? That is because the side effects of those drugs are still present in your body. They need to be alleviated with just another pill.

So if you are feeling stressed out and you want to reach for a drug which you think is going to relax you, my immediate suggestion is – Stop That Immediately.

Read this instead –

Question – Why Are You Taking This Drug?

Your answer – because I feel stressed out and I want to relax.

Q – So you think that taking the drug is going to stop you from being stressed out.

YA – yes, and if it cannot do that, at least, it will relax me. I am so tense. I am really stressed out. I need that drug. I need to relax.

Q – So you think that that drug is helping you to relax? What makes you think that?

YA [a bit exasperated] I told you I am stressed out. I really have no patience with your damn fool questions. I need that drug. I really do not want a lecture on why I am taking this drug. I am taking it to feel relaxed. You are not helping my tense state. If I do not take that drug, I will not feel relaxed. My stressed-out condition will worsen. And that will be because of you, because you are asking me silly questions instead of allowing me to take that drug.

Q – Have you heard yourself speak? You sound almost frantic and desperate. You say you are stressed out and that is why you want to take that drug. You think that that is going to help you relax. Do not you feel that you are addicted to that drug, and believe that it is the only way in which you can relax? Do not you think that this sounds perilously close to dependence on a drug?

YA(extremely indignant) do not be silly! There is no question of my ever being addicted to anything, as you say it. I am an extremely responsible person, and there is no way in which I will allow myself to be addicted to anything. That drug was prescribed to me by a doctor. He said that it would help me relax. It is helping me relax. It is helping me from being stressed out. It is helping me from getting tense.

Q-Do you really think so?

YA- I NEED MY MEDICINE! You stop hounding me. Just Get lost, I really do not have the time to listen to your futile burbling, you interfering busybody, you. I know what I am doing and I could do without your advice. Thank you for nothing. [and other associated bad tempered statements…]

Now, if you ever found yourself in this situation [God forbid] and you have read the above dialogue, is not it time you faced the facts?

Drugs are used as a last resort to alleviate a painful and chronic physical illness to help heal the body. On the other hand, just popping drugs, thinking that they are going to help relax you, especially when you are stressed, is definitely not healthy. Nor is it advisable. That means you do not intend to cure you of stress and tension. When you have a drug handy, it is going to do the job for you. You know the right pill to pop whenever you feel stressed. And that pill makes you feel really good. It gives you this feeling of euphoria. You really cannot do without it.

And then just imagine, there comes a time when you cannot get this pill. Disaster, despair, desperation. You are all stressed out because you have not got a pill which helps you relax. Why take it in the first place?

Instead, try some other natural stress busters, of which I am going to tell you more in the next chapter.

Yoga – The Best Stress Buster and Meditation

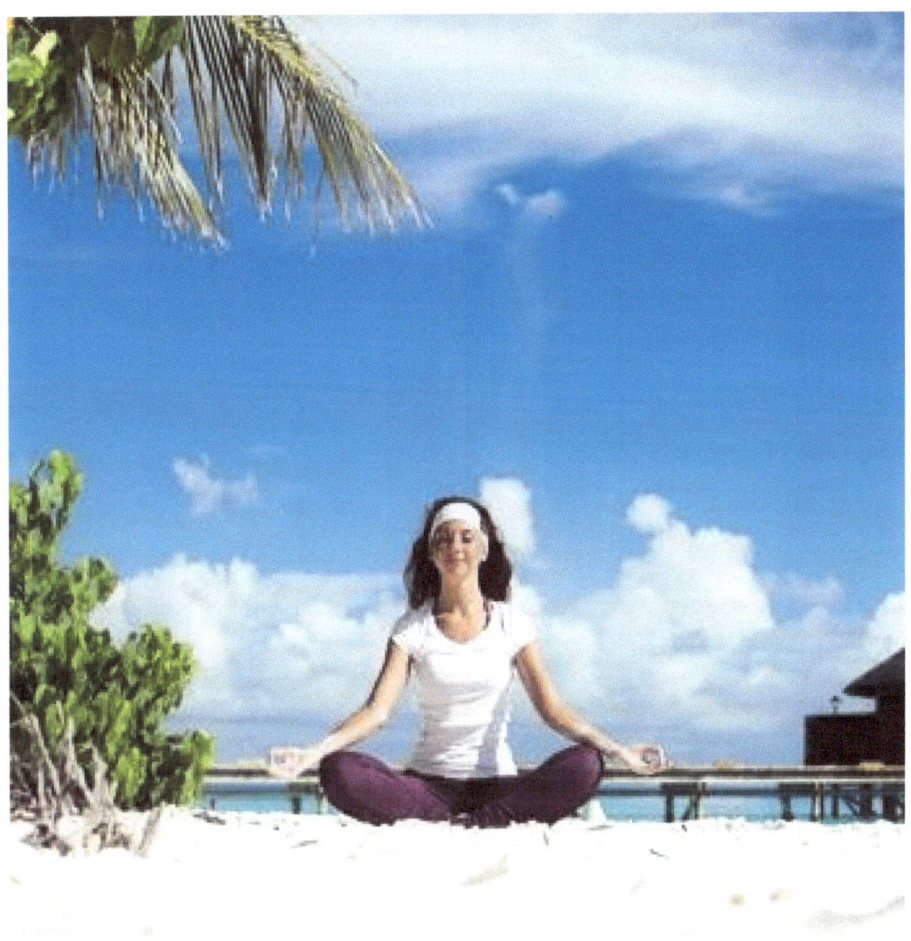

I am not promoting yoga, just because it is a part of the social, cultural and traditional of my country, but because I know that it is a part of the ancient way of living. Yoga is a teaching which does not belong to any one people, tribe, country or religion; instead, it is universal, and this knowledge has been used for millenniums by people who want to achieve physical, spiritual, emotional and mental harmony.

I asked an American friend of mine about 20 years ago to try yoga for beating stress. His immediate reaction was, "hey, is not that something preached by the Hindus in India. You had to do religious chants when you are practicing yoga exercises." He did not intend to sit in a lotus pose chanting Om and other chants. He did not intend to do that ever."

Seriously, having lived in India and having yoga such an integral part of my daily life, I did not know that some people believed that this was the religious prerogative of just the Hindus and one had to chant Om and also prayers. I had to gain that bit of knowledge from a Western friend! So I kept quiet. Luckily, another Hindu friend enlightened him. Now that person knew everything about yoga. From him the both of us got to know that chanting that particular word was a necessary part of yoga is a misconception, – though it helps to focus one's mind while meditating –. The idea that chanting religious *shlokas* while meditating was something promulgated later on, down the road, by some misguided people who intended to corner the credit for knowledge, which was gathered by the wise ancients to help mankind.

Yoga is universal. It is for everyone. These ancients who gathered the knowledge brought to you from yoga did not bother about who you were and who you worshipped; they just intended for you to benefit from their teachings. They were spiritually too highly evolved and were above the petty earth bound considerations of caste, creed and religion. They intended to benefit the future generations of mankind regardless of color, race, and belief.

Besides, the word AUM is not restricted to just the Hindus. The Buddhists chant *Om name Padme hum* when they are meditating. This word is not restricted to one religion, but is considered to be the universal Alpha of the beginning of all things. This word is supposed to be a powerful way in which to call on the powers of the universe in order to relieve stress, strain, and tension. It is helping you to reach the state of mental, physical and spiritual harmony with the elements around you. You are garnering everything that is good, which is around you and which you can get through a little bit of meditation and yoga. And thanks to the West opening up to the spiritual, mental and physical benefits of yoga in the late 90s, it has begun to be a universal boon to mankind.

Yoga was the way of life in the Indian subcontinent since prehistoric times, even before people began to think of the concept of religion and beliefs. This idea was how to work for the good of everyone around you. The religious books and teachings garnered by these wise men are now a very sacred and integral part of Hindu tradition and its religion, but their main aim was to benefit every living soul out there.

Thus my friend's hesitation about taking up yoga – though valid and justified in his mind, because he is a religious person, –was explained properly by a sensible and very knowledgeable yogi.

I am not a Hindu. I am not a Buddhist. I am a chronically stressed sentient carbon based human being. Sometimes I Chant Om and sometimes I just make a continuous low pitched humming noise deep in my throat while breathing in deeply. If it sounds nasal and more of a low HMMMMMMMM sound that does not worry me. Because my job is to get rid of stress, and not get entangled with any controversial potentially stress making trivialities, which may prevent you and me from gaining the harmonious and knowledgeable benefits brought to us by the ancients.

Also, that low noise in my throat is the best way in which I can get rid of my hypothyroidism because the vibrations stimulate the thalamus! Now this is yoga at its very best!

So how do you benefit from yoga?

You have to be in a state of mind in which you want to relax. If you think that you can relax when you are going to be interrupted by your schedule Alarm going off in the next 30 minutes , so that you are in time for an important meeting, I would suggest you postpone your session. There are 10 minute meditation tapes, which can help and relax you. They are good to relieve stress, but 30 minutes from now, you are going to go straight into stress mode again. So you need permanent solutions on how to counteract stress.

If you have a garden near you, how lucky you are. You can just go and sit down on the lawn and take deep breaths of fresh oxygen. Look around you. Concentrate on what you are looking at instead of allowing your mind to think while your eyes focus on something without really "seeing" that. Then close your eyes. Allow your body to relax. If you are an action based person, this is something which is not going to come natural to you. Such people cannot relax. Then take deep breaths. Visualize a lamp glowing. Concentrate on it. Or just say the 23rd Psalm, take the name of Allah or the God in which you believe or just say Aum or any power word which you consider to be an affirmation of life, power, and universal harmony. Just thinking that word or saying a prayer helps in combating stress. That is because you are trying to reaffirm your belief that everything is going to turn out right, and you have faith in the higher powers that they are going to give you the best help and guidance in helping you solve your problems.

Once you have decided that you have meditated enough and find yourself relax, get up and tackle those problems. God is not going to help you, if you keep saying, help me, help me, but do not make the effort to do something affirmation and constructive.

This reminds me of an old chestnut – there was this person who had faith and a firm belief that whatever he wished for would be granted. Now this was positive thinking of a superior kind. So he kept praying to win the multimillion dollar jackpot. And the result came out. He had not won it. Indignantly, he spoke to God –"here was I expecting to win this jackpot and here I thought that you would help me win that jackpot. Why did you not do that?" And God answered him, "how could I do so when you did not buy a lottery ticket in the first place?"

So if you are thinking that your problems are going to be solved by just wishing that they would go away, that is not going to happen. You need mental, emotional, spiritual and physical strength in order to tackle them. And you will soon find that they are not as insurmountable as you thought, because you are facing reality and you have the strength to tackle all your problems.

Problem-Solving and How That Helps You Cope with Stress

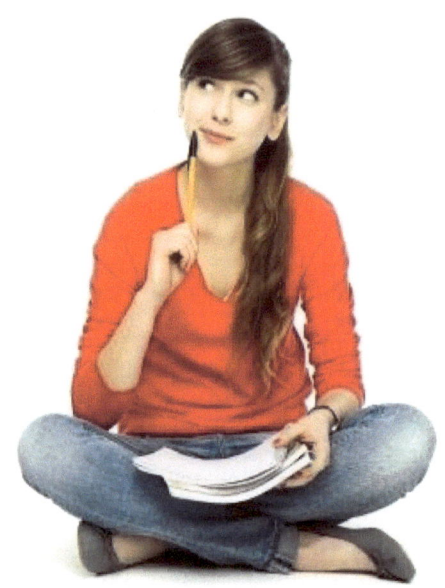

One of the more negative side effects of stress is that your problem-solving capacities are diminished. You find you not capable of making a decision for even trivial matters. You find yourself procrastinating. You find yourself wondering about why you cannot make such an easy decision and give someone a final answer. You find yourself vacillating between decisions. This makes you feel tense. What is happening to you? Why cannot you make a decision? Are you losing your decision-making and problem-solving capacities? Well, you are well on your way to becoming a stressed person.

So if you are stressed, just because you cannot make decisions right now, here are some tips and techniques in which you can solve your problems.

Take some time off because you are going to concentrate on your problems and the reasons why you are so stressed out.

Take a pen and paper. Now start listing out all the reasons which you think that are potential stress making factors. They can be anything ranging from financial problems to personal health problems, problems of relationships, professional problems, and any other thing that comes to mind. The bigger the list is, the more things you will be able to tackle, when you are getting your mind to concentrate on these tension building factors and reasons.

In fact, I found one woman got stressed out because she was obsessive about cleanliness and according to her her husband still treated the house as a bachelor pad. She was tired of picking and carrying after him. She was really stressed out. I told her why she thought that this was the reason which made her tense. Was not he a good husband and father? Had not he been a responsible provider for his family Lo these many years? Did not he worked hard all hours of the day, earning money for her and her children to spend in riotous living, and even then, she still considered that he did not have the right to come back home after a hard day's work and take off his shoes in the living room. That caused her stress. She was a selfish, self-indulgent spoiled female.

She blinked when she heard me say all that. How could I call her selfish? She spent all her day keeping the house immaculate. She was so proud of her home and garden. Her whole identity was tied up with it. That in itself caused her so much stress. He should at least respect the effort to go on into that activity, and take off the shoes in the bedroom.

I decided that this female was going to be stressed, for absolutely no reason whatsoever, and if she did not have any reason, she would invent one. There are many people out there like her. They are so absolutely bored doing nothing, or something they consider to be the be-all and end-all of their existence and because they have nothing really constructive to do that they invent reasons to get stressed.

Now if she went out in the real world and did an honest day's work just like her husband did, she would get to face reality. He had more reasons for being stressed. He had the responsibility of coming home to a whining woman who really did not make him welcome, but was more bothered about what her neighbors would say, if there was a speck of dust on the top of her cupboards. I believe this behavior to be obsessive and neurotic. This sort of woman will not be able to solve any of her problems because she does not have the mental capacity or the ability or the will or the inclination to find a really good solution to why she is stressed. It takes one second to pick up a pair of shoes. But she would rather indulge in 35 minutes of complaining. I think that that was wasted time, and there are so many time wasters out there who would rather talk than do something constructive in order to solve their problems.

Sensible people look more into problem-solving than wasting their time procrastinating. So now that you have a list of all your problems put them under different headings.

What are the things I cannot help?

These may be tension making problems, like personal commitments or getting stressed because of ill health in the family. These may be unsolvable or they may have a solution. If you cannot solve them, like you cannot do anything if someone died, getting stressed about this factor is unreasonable. Now if that person's death has caused plenty of problems for you, including personal, financial and emotional problems, this is when you need to look at the next point –

What are the things that I can solve?

Now these are some things which may take plenty of time and effort to solve. Most of your stress is caused by the feeling that you may not have the physical, emotional, spiritual, or even financial strength to solve these problems. But once you have faced these problems squarely, you will notice that many of them were not so serious as you thought they were in the first place. In fact, you may find some problems extremely trivial when compared to larger problems. So cross them out. You will find your list being reduced drastically.

So perhaps you started with 15 to 20 potentially stress making factors in the first place. You cross out the ones which you think trivial. You cross out the ones which you cannot help and which come under the category of "act of nature", and which is a part of life-and-death. You are soon going to find that although potential stress making problems have been reduced drastically to just a few major factors. And these are the ones with which you have to deal for the rest of your life.

Now the best example of problem solving can be seen in a story told about Alexander. He heard about the Gordian knot and how it had been tied by an ancient named Gordius. Ancient legends supposedly said that anybody who unraveled the Gordian knot would conquer the world. Many warriors had tried to do that but they could not do it. Alexander went straight up to the knot, took out his sword and cut it into two. There, it had been unraveled. Now he was not using common methods of problem solving, he just thought of something which no one had thought before. Now he was someone who applied his brains in thinking and solving a problem. And being a showman, he solved the problem of the Gordian knot in the most melodramatic method of which he could think. And that made his soldiers believe that he was fated to conquer the world. Well, talk about psychology!

Let me give you another example of thinking out of the box, in rather more modern times. There is a world-famous iron pillar erected by the Emperor Asoka,(named the Great 250 BCE) in the area surrounding Kutub Minar in Delhi. Ancient legend says that anybody who can encircle the pillar – with his back touching the surface of the pillar – and gets his hands to clasp each other in a fist will conquer the world. Fate has deemed him a *Chakravarty*. The legend also said that this encircling of the pillar with long arms and long fingered hands could only be done by Asoka – who was the *Chakravarty Samraat* or world conqueror of his time and age, and the pillar's girth was made accordingly.

The girth of the pillar is such that 99.99 percent of the people cannot do that. But I knew how to tackle that problem and being a bit of a show off and limelight grabber myself in my salad days, I used to go to that pillar and see people trying desperately hard to clasp their hands behind them and making a fist. And I would go marching up – to the tune of an imaginary fanfare, look at my audience for a couple of seconds and then with a deep puff of breath exhaled through my nose- do that easily, to the astonishment, bewilderment, and wonder of the tourists and visitors there.

Now how did I do that? I noticed that it was easier for a person to clasp one's hands together if he lifted up his hands and clasped them about his head or around his shoulder region *where the iron pillar was less thick in girth*. Everybody naturally tried to clasp their arms and palms around their waist region. So voila, I with my long anthropoidal arms and talon like claws could do that easily and there was everybody, looking wide-eyed and asking their family to "Look, look, look, she, standing there, she can encircle the pillar, she can and will conquer the world one day because she is born a *Chakravartini*."[1]

So simple when you think about it, is not it. A little bit of applied logic, and plenty of fun as a result.

I do not intend to be a world conqueror. It is too stress making, and is best left to people with lots of ambition and people who like being stressed! But the point of this story is, there is absolutely nothing in the world which

---

[1] Incidentally, I asked a historian friend about this legend, of which he knew. And I told him that I could do that encircling bit and I also admitted about how I managed to do it. He looked at me for a couple of seconds and then told me, very gravely and frankly, "do you know, when we were doing some work in that area, all of us tried tackling that pillar. And we also lifted up our hands to shoulder level like you say you did and tried making our joined hands in a fist. None of us could do so. 99.99% of the people I know cannot do that, even when they try lifting their hands to shoulder level. So tell me when you decide to conquer the world so that I can be your historian. That is what the second part of the ancient legend says – nobody can escape his fate. The pillar foretold your fate for you and you can do absolutely nothing about it. If it is written, it is written. "That last bit about fate left me blinking. Whether he was pulling my leg about the conquer the world Bit and also a ruthless fate, nobody can say with these serious academics, can one. But I intend to do absolutely nothing. I am not buying any lottery tickets to give fate a chance to put me into a stress building lifestyle, yet, once again! Been there seen that.

cannot be solved without a bit of thinking out of the box. Also, you need to be able to laugh at yourself, at the world around you, and at the present simplicity of everything in life!

Conclusion

So now you know all about stress and tension, the reasons for stress, and its possible side effects, factors causing the stress and how to tackle them through problem-solving or just a little bit of common sense and thinking outside the box, remember that there is absolutely no problem in the world – apart from those beyond our control – for which there is not some solution somewhere. So if you find yourself stressed out, and your life full of Tension, the tips and techniques given in this book are going to help you a lot, I hope.

Believe it or not, 121 million people all over the globe suffer from depression. A majority of these patients' condition was aggravated because they had no support when they were undergoing stress. 77% of people in the USA suffer from stress, which can lead to depression. So if you feel stressed, do talk about this with your friends, and your doctor. Also, I would suggest a bit of discernment here. If you are a compulsive worry wart and go broadcasting your problems to all your friends at the drop of a hat, and exaggerating them out of all proportion, it will be a situation of "cry Wolf" when you really find yourself stressed. Nobody is going to help you then because they are going to consider you really seriously suffering from stress when you are justified in asking for help and support.

Remember that a little bit of stress is a part of everyone's daily life, but if you allow it to take over your life, you need help fast. So best of luck and the power of harmony and good go with you.

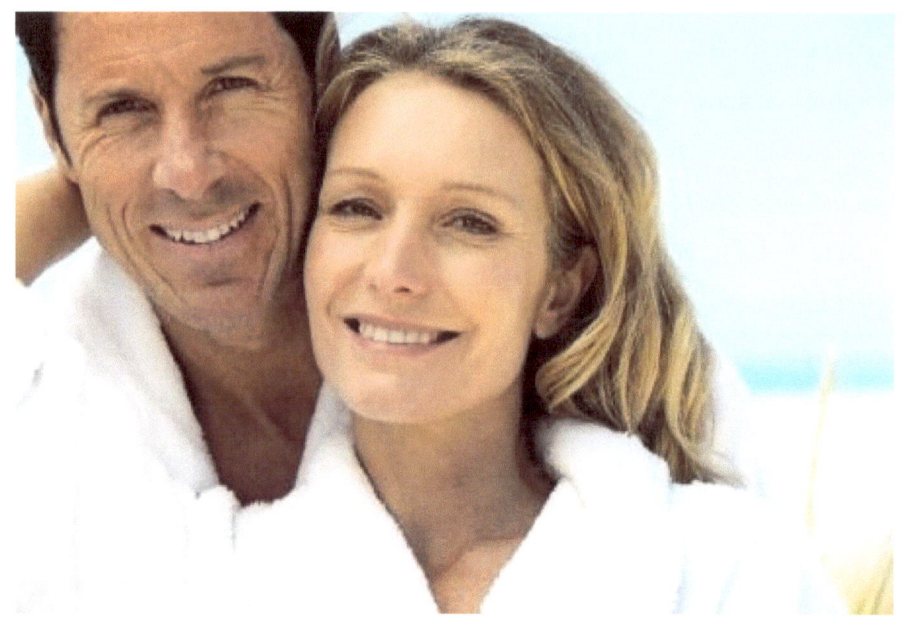

Live life Emperor size sans stress sans tension.

Author Bio

Dueep Jyot Singh is a Management and IT Professional who managed to gather Postgraduate qualifications in Management and English and Degrees in Science, French and Education while pursuing different enjoyable career options like being an hospital administrator, IT,SEO and HRD Database Manager/ trainer, movie scriptwriter, theatre artiste and public speaker, lecturer in French, Marketing and Advertising, ex-Editor of Hearts On Fire (now known as Solctice) Books Missouri USA, advice columnist and cartoonist, publisher and Aviation School trainer, ex- moderator on Medico.in, banker, student councilor ,travelogue writer … among other things! One fine morning, she decided that she had enough of killing herself by Degrees and went back to her first love -- writing. It's more enjoyable! She already has 24 published academic and 11 fiction- in- different- genre books under her belt.

When she is not designing websites or making Graphic design illustrations for clients who want Walt Disney, Norman Rockwell , JJ Grandville or Hed Kandy type illustrations, she is busy browsing in old bookshops for antique books,-she has a mouthwatering collection of priceless First editions and rare books…including R.L. Stevenson, O.Henry, Dornford Yates, Maurice Walsh, C.N.Williamson, and the crown of her collection- Dickens "The Old Curiosity Shop," and so on… Just call her "Renaissance Woman") - collecting herbal remedies, making one of a kind creations in Irish Crochet and Aran knitting, acting like Universal Helping Hand/Agony Aunt, or escaping to her dear mountains for a bit of exploring, collecting herbs and plants , trekking and rappelling.

Check out some of the other JD-Biz Publishing books

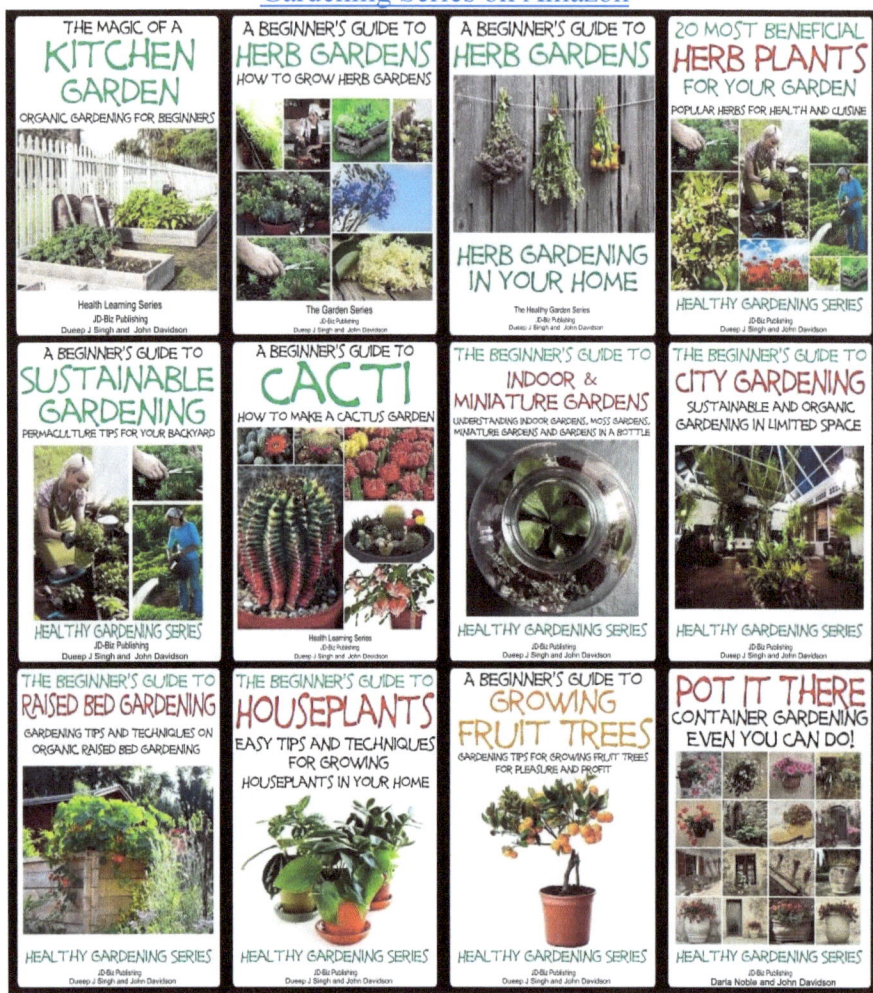

Download Free Books!

http://MendonCottageBooks.com

Health Learning Series

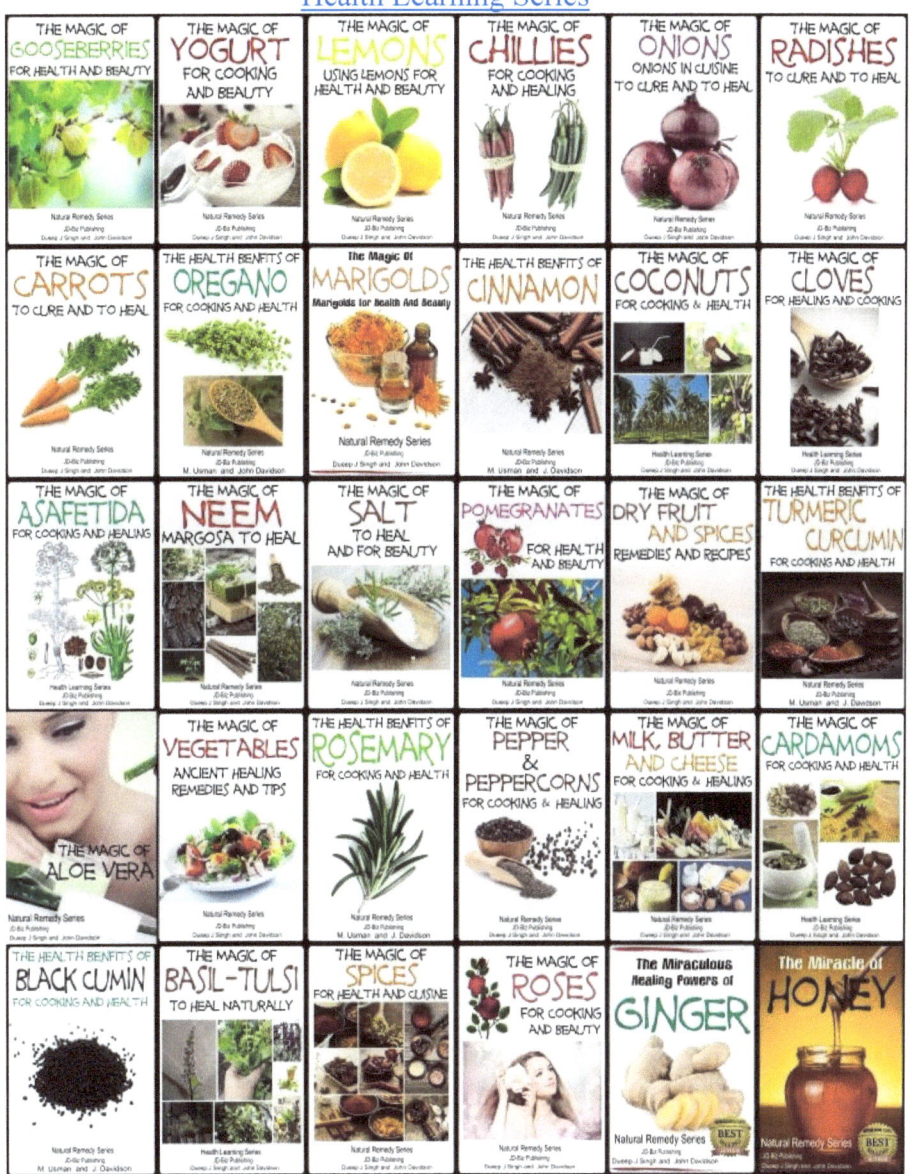

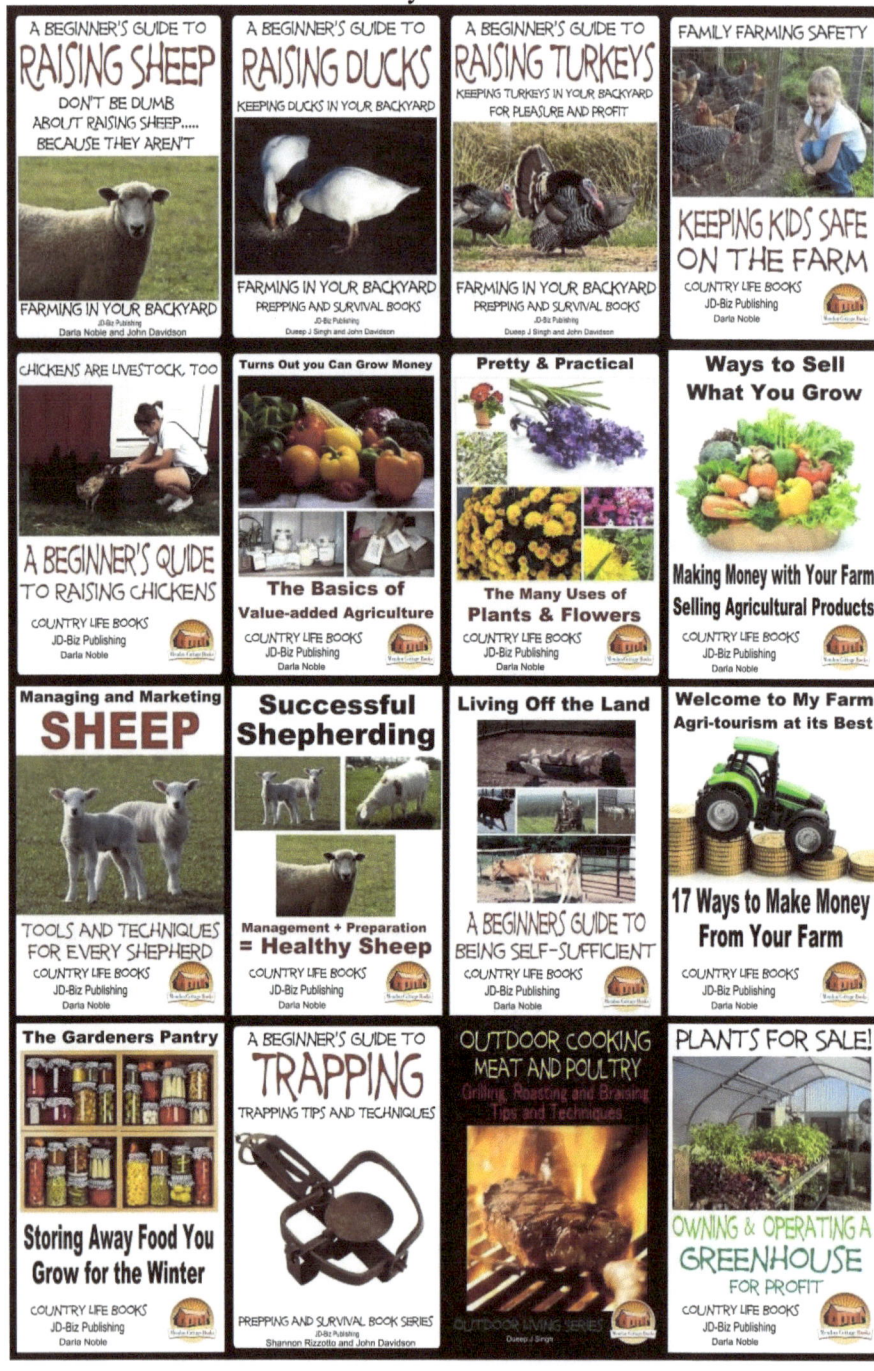

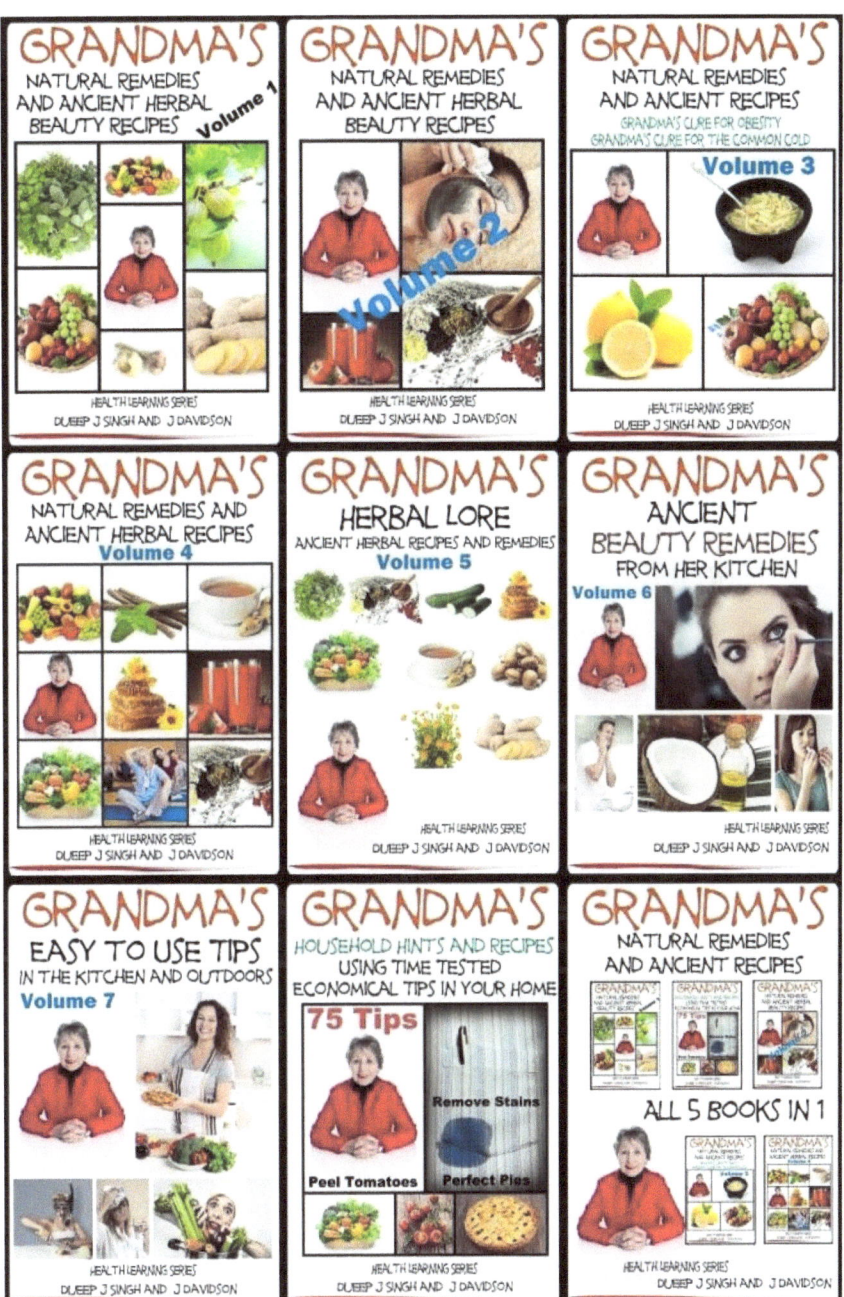

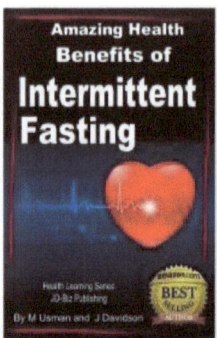
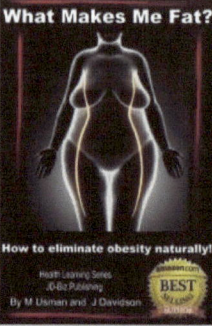
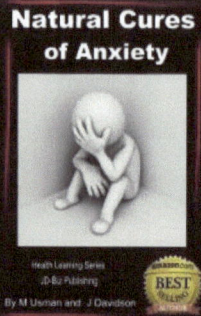
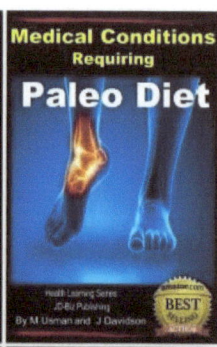

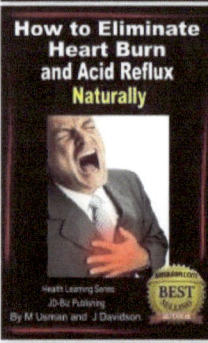
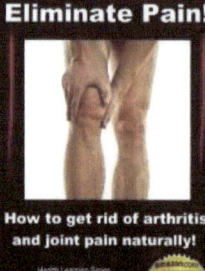
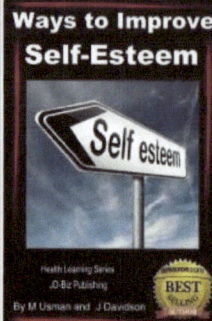
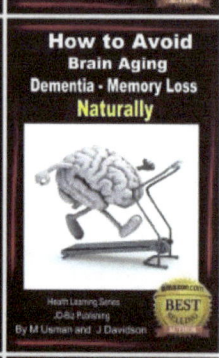

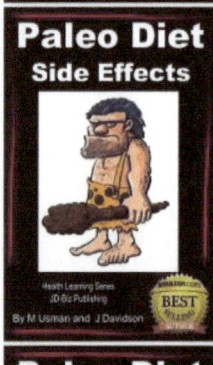
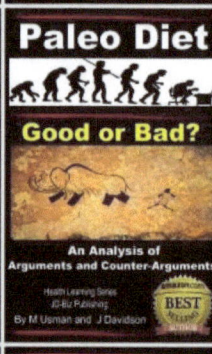
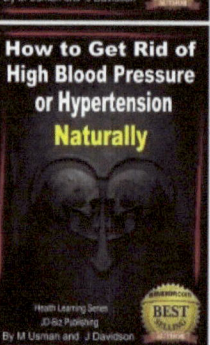
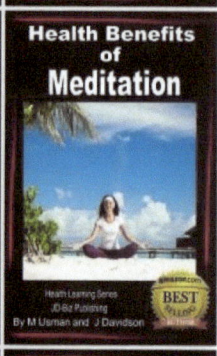

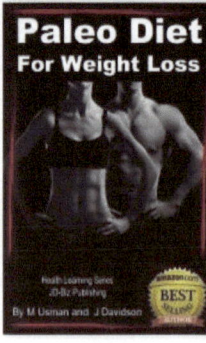
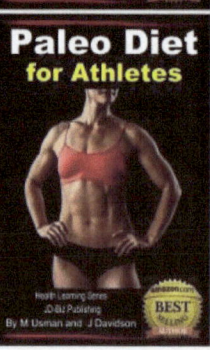
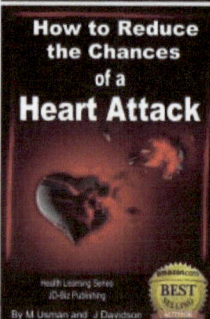
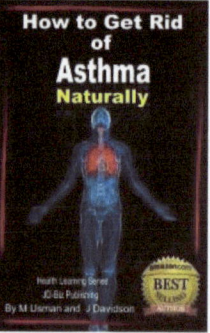

Amazing Animal Book Series

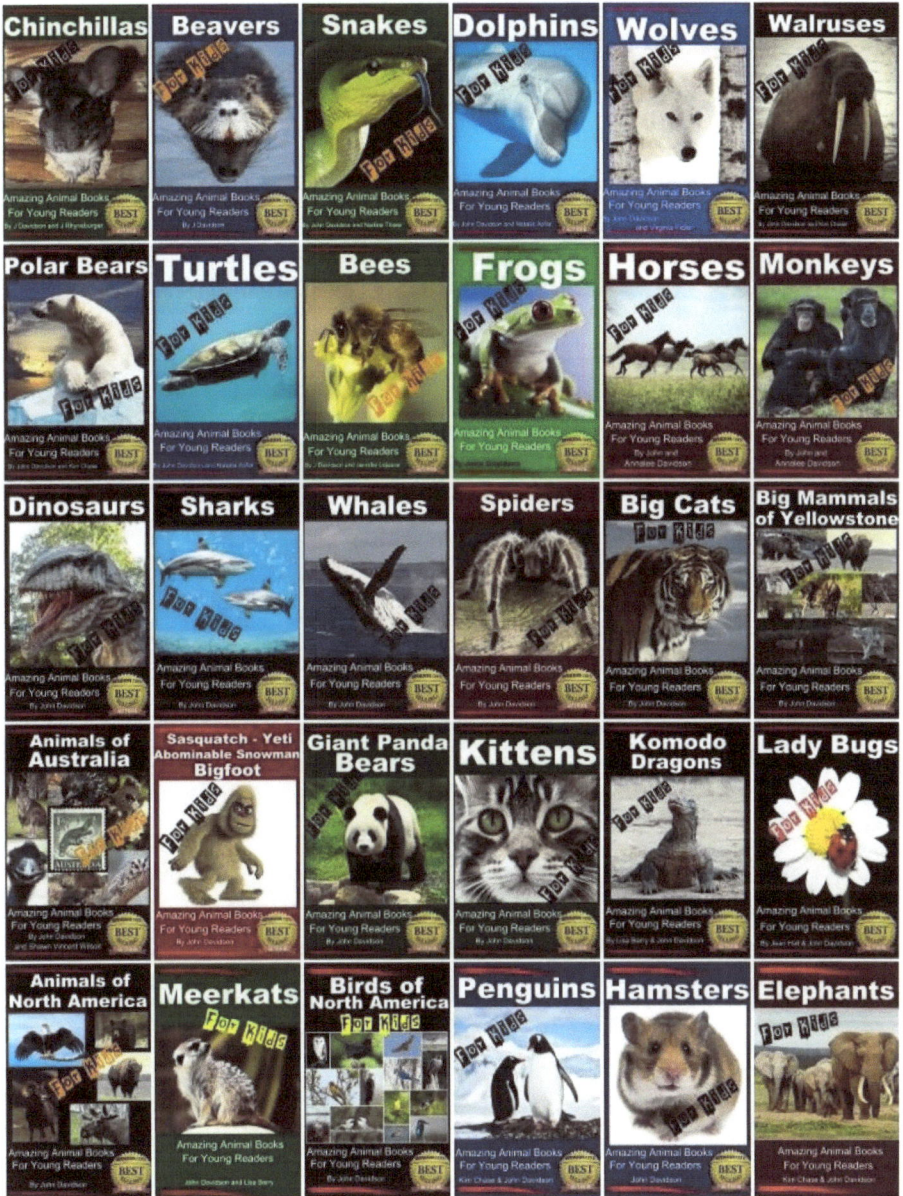

Learn To Draw Series

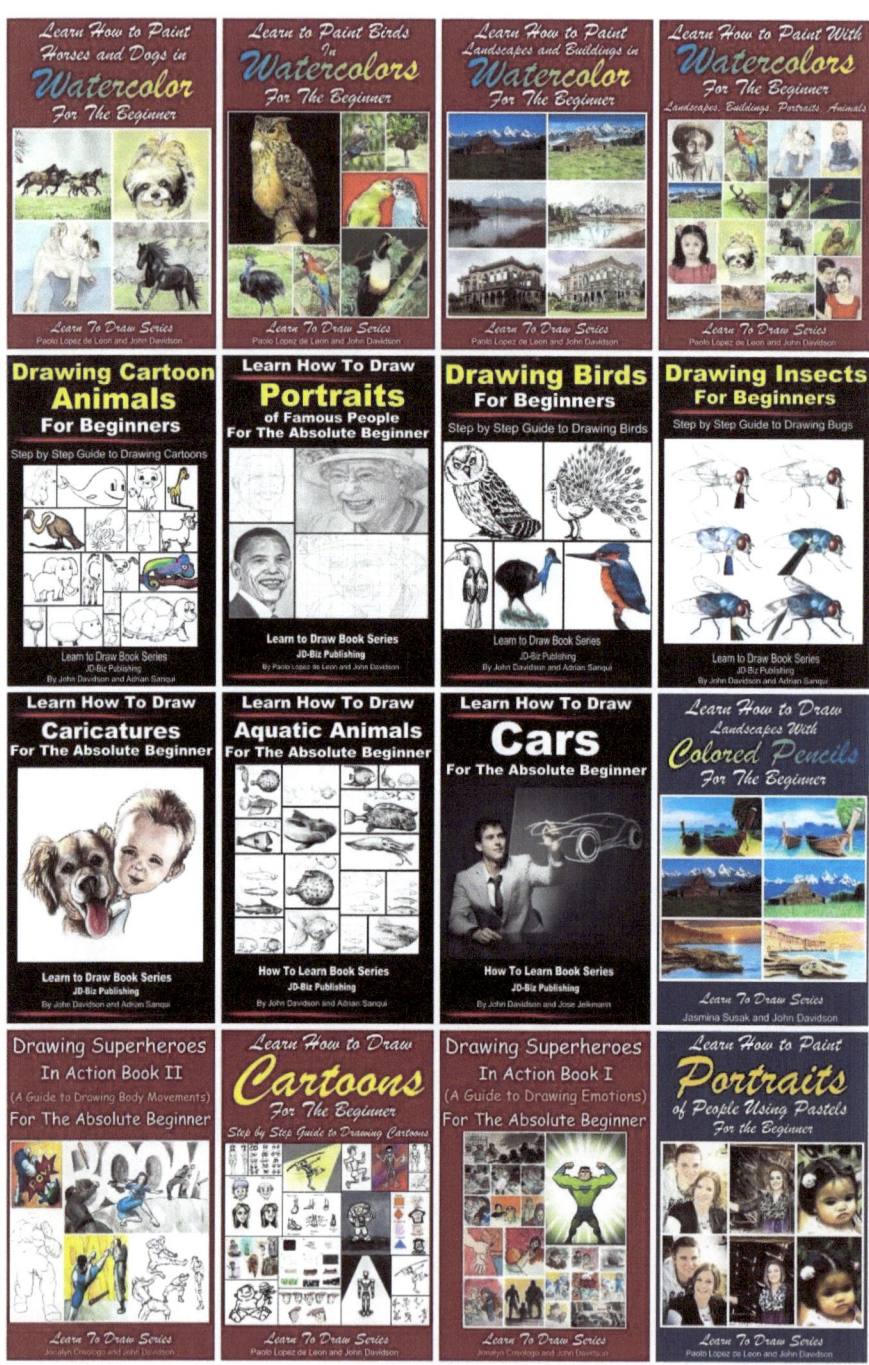

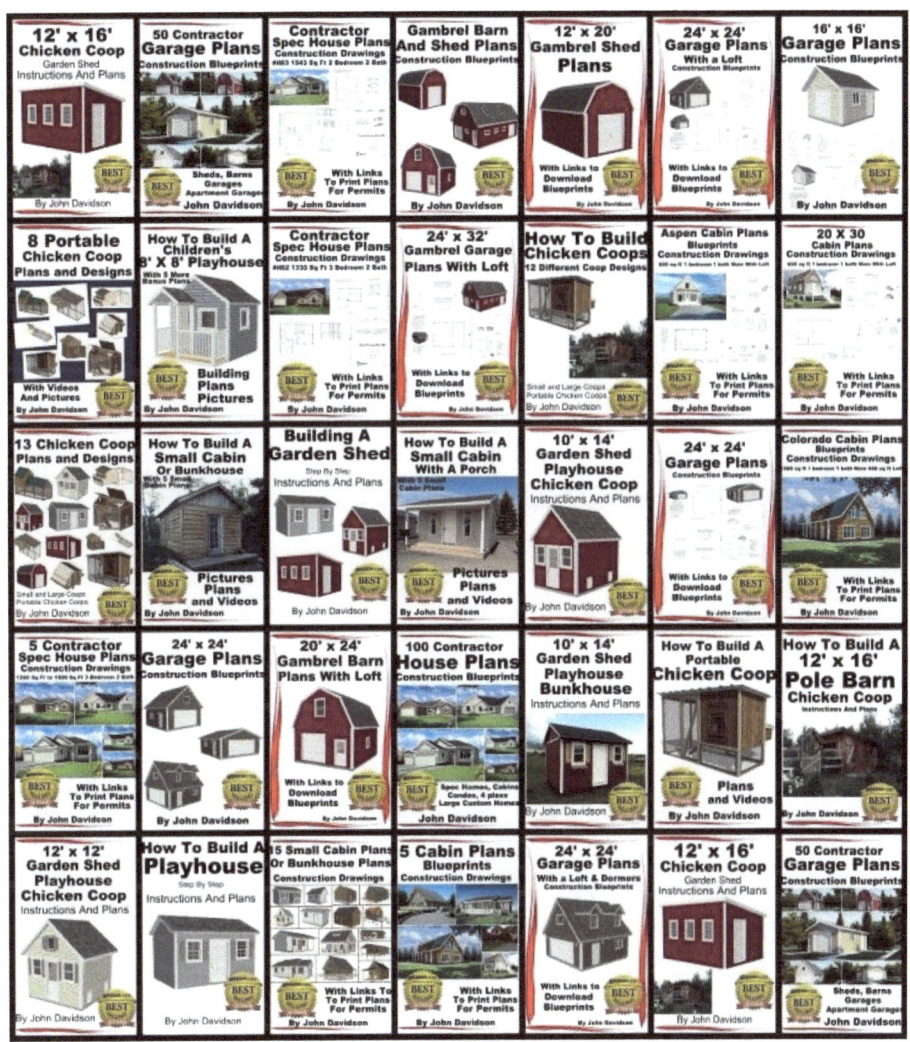

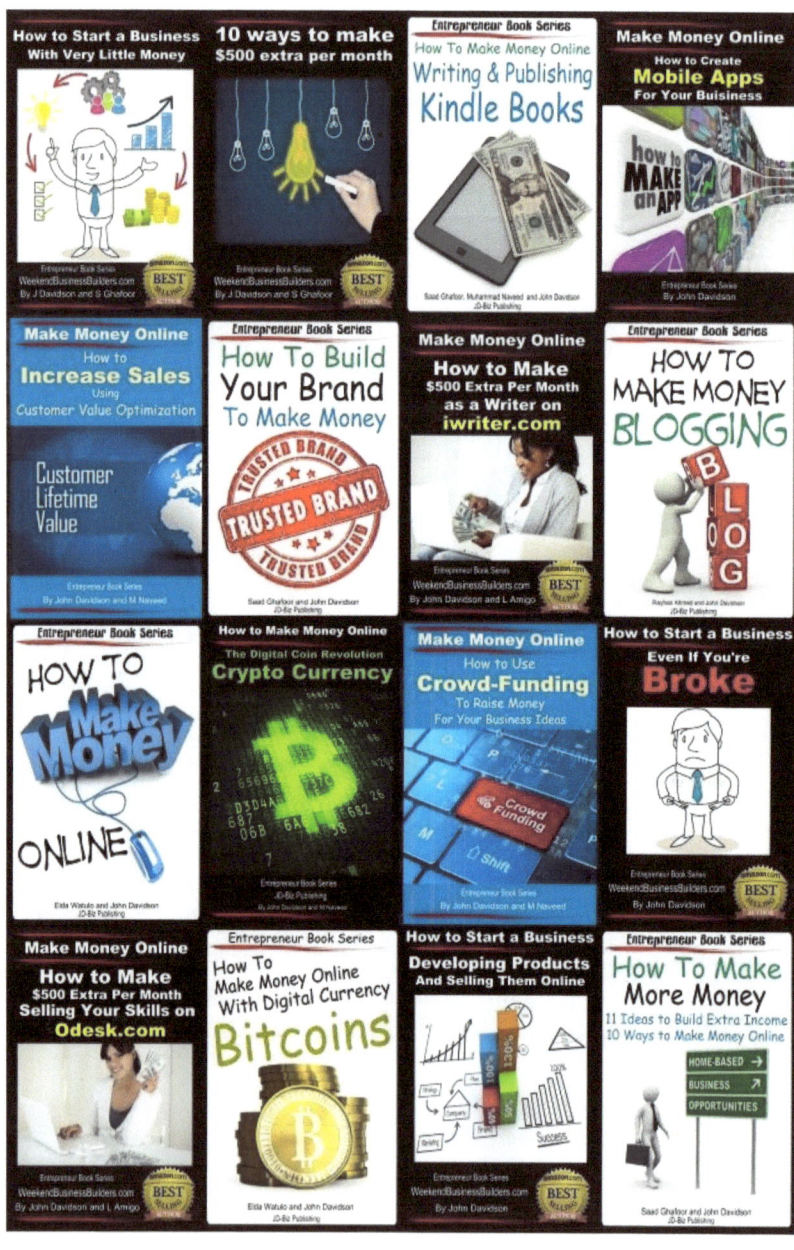

Our books are available at

1. Amazon.com
2. Barnes and Noble
3. Itunes
4. Kobo
5. Smashwords
6. Google Play Books

Download Free Books!

http://MendonCottageBooks.com

Publisher

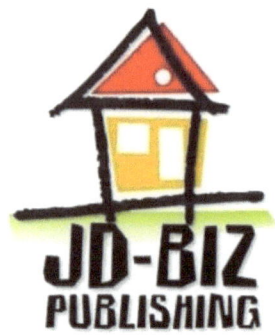

JD-Biz Corp

P O Box 374

Mendon, Utah 84325

http://www.jd-biz.com/

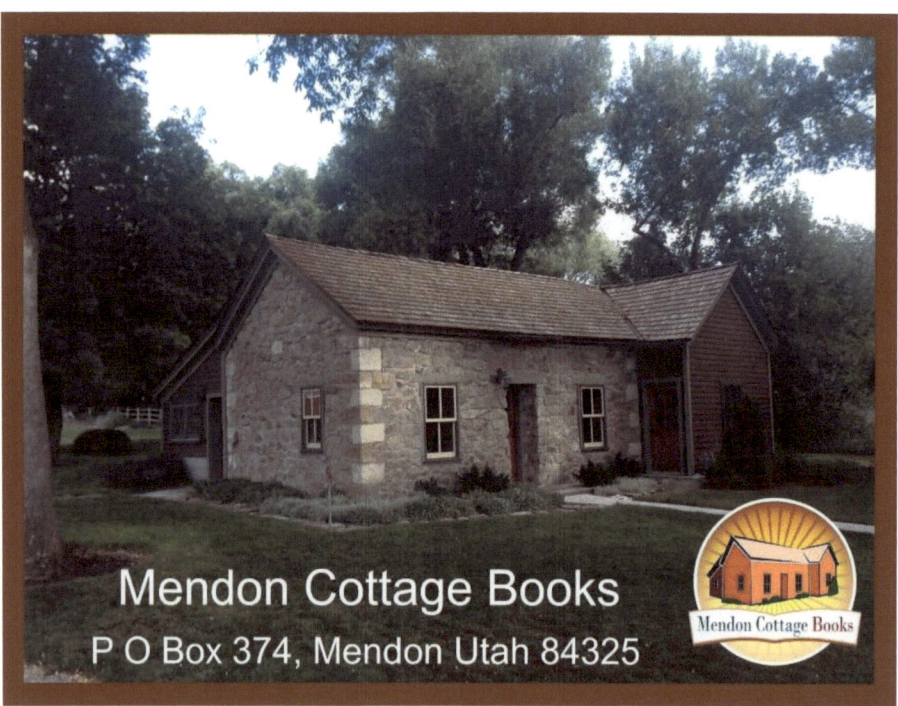

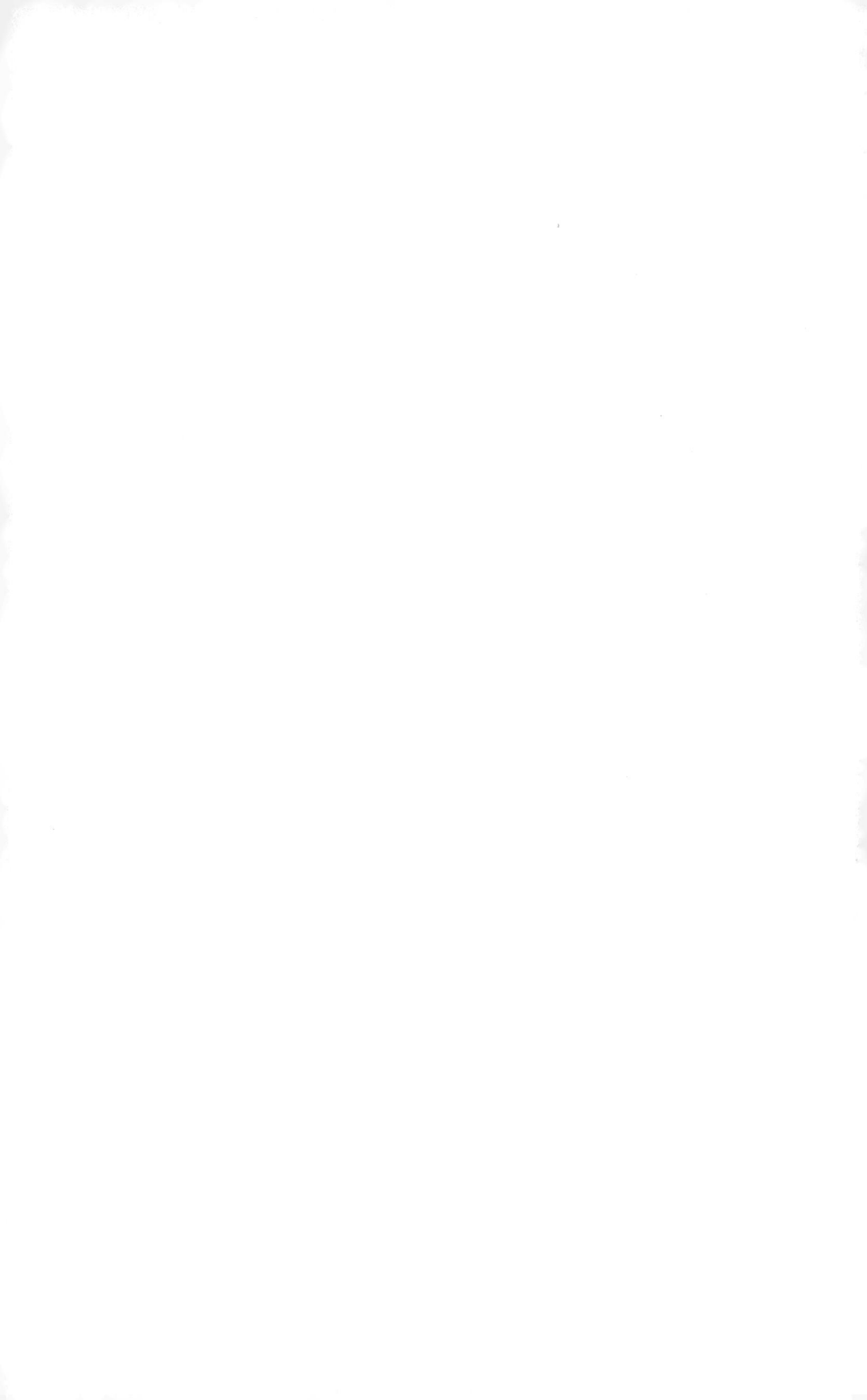